the Unofficial Guide™ to Overcoming Infertility

Joan Liebmann-Smith, Ph.D.,
Jacqueline Nardi Egan, and
John Stangel, M.D.

Macmillan • USA

O9-AIG-685

Macmillan General Reference
A Pearson Education Macmillan Company
1633 Broadway
New York, New York 10019-6785

ISBN: 0-02-862916-7

Manufactured in the United States of America

10 9 8 7 6 5 4 3 2 1

First edition

*This book is dedicated to my husband, Richard, and
my daughter, Rebecca, for all their love and support
and for their understanding of all the late hours
and missed meals.*

—Joan Liebmann-Smith, Ph.D.

*This book is dedicated to my husband, Edward, for his
unfailing support and strength; and to our daughter,
Elizabeth, for her encouragement and enthusiasm.*

—Jacqueline Nardi Egan

*To Lois, Eric and Justin with love and appreciation. To
my patients, who have shared their problems and feelings
with me, who have taught more than any textbook, and
who have allowed me the privilege of treating them. To
those who yearn to have a child of their own, I wish you
the fulfillment of your dreams.*

—John Stangel, M.D.

*The authors would also like to dedicate this book to their
friends, relatives, and all the six million American couples who are faced with infertility.*

Acknowledgments

First and foremost we'd like to thank our co-author, Dr. John Stangel, for his expertise, contributions, suggestions and advice on all aspects of this book. We'd also like to thank Dr. Loren Greene, who introduced us to Macmillan's *Unofficial* series, and Dr. Sami David and Dr. Harris Nagler for their careful reading of the manuscript, and helpful comments and suggestions. Special thanks to Dr. Alan Trounson of Monash University, Dr. Robert Visscher, former executive director of the American Society for Reproductive Medicine (ASRM) and Dr. Larry Lipshultz, president of ASRM, for taking the time to provide us with their insights about the current state and future direction of infertility treatment. Sean Tipton and Heather Kowalski, also of ASRM, and Joyce Zeitz of the Society for Assisted Reproductive Technology, provided us with invaluable information, data and other resources.

Dianne Aronson and Dianne Clapp, RN, of RESOLVE, were extremely helpful in getting us pertinent information in a moment's notice. We also want to thank RESOLVE itself for being there as a terrific resource, not only for us writers, but more importantly, for the millions of people struggling with infertility.

Many thanks to Leslie Nies of Serono Symposia; and Gary Weinberg, Barry Nysenbaum, Joseph Gennardo and Jack Cody of Park Avenue Chemists (aka Boghan Pharmacy), for providing educational materials, books and brochures on infertility to us, as well as infertile patients.

Thanks to all the Jennifers and Nancys past and present at Macmillan, especially Jennifer Perillo, managing editor of the *Unofficial Guides* and Nancy Gratton, our development editor. Jennifer has been a Guardian Angel—her professionalism, attention to detail, and sanity in the sometimes insane world of publishing have been beyond the call. We couldn't have done this without her support and help. Nancy's unfailing encouragement, and calm, reassuring attitude got us through many crises.

And last but not least, we wish to thank Richard and Rebecca Liebmann-Smith, and Edward and Elizabeth Egan for their continued love, support and understanding especially during our marathon work sessions.

Joan Liebmann-Smith, Ph.D.

Jacqueline Nardi Egan

Contents

The *Unofficial Guide* Reader's Bill of Rights

We Give You More Than the Official Line

Welcome to the *Unofficial Guide* series of Lifestyles titles—books that deliver critical, unbiased information that other books can't or won't reveal—*the inside scoop*. Our goal is to provide you with the *most accessible, useful* information and advice possible. The recommendations we offer in these pages are not influenced by the corporate line of any organization or industry; we give you the hard facts, whether those institutions like them or not. If something is ill-advised or will cause a loss of time and/or money, we'll give you ample warning. And if it is a worthwhile option, we'll let you know that, too.

Armed and Ready

Our hand-picked authors confidently and critically report on a wide range of topics that matter to smart readers like you. Our authors are passionate about their subjects, but have distanced themselves enough from them to help you be armed and protected, and help you make educated decisions as you go through your process. It is our intent that, from having read this book, you will avoid the pitfalls everyone else falls into and get it right the first time.

Don't be fooled by cheap imitations; this is the genuine article *Unofficial Guide* series from Macmillan Publishing. You may be familiar with our proven track record of the travel *Unofficial Guides,* which have more than three million copies in print. Each year thousands of travelers—new and old—are armed with a brand new, fully updated edition of the flagship *Unofficial Guide to Walt Disney World,* by Bob Sehlinger. It is our intention here to provide you with the same level of objective authority that Mr. Sehlinger does in his brainchild.

The Unofficial Panel of Experts

Every work in the Lifestyle *Unofficial Guides* is intensively inspected by a team of top professionals in their fields. These experts review the manuscript for factual accuracy, comprehensiveness, and an insider's determination as to whether the manuscript fulfills the credo in this Reader's Bill of Rights. In other words, our Panel ensures that you are, in fact, getting "the inside scoop."

Our Pledge

The authors, the editorial staff, and the Unofficial Panel of Experts assembled for *Unofficial Guides* are determined to lay out the most valuable alternatives available for our readers. This dictum means that our writers must be explicit, prescriptive, and above all, direct. We strive to be thorough and complete, but our goal is not necessarily to have the "most" or "all" of the information on a topic; this is not, after all, an encyclopedia. Our objective is to help you narrow down your options to the best of what is available, unbiased by affiliation with any industry or organization.

In each *Unofficial Guide* we give you:

- Comprehensive coverage of necessary and vital information

- Authoritative, rigidly fact-checked data

- The most up-to-date insights into trends

- Savvy, sophisticated writing that's also readable

- Sensible, applicable facts and secrets that only an insider knows

Special Features

Every book in our series offers the following six special sidebars in the margins that were devised to help you get things done cheaply, efficiently, and smartly.

1. "Timesaver"—tips and shortcuts that save you time.

2. "Moneysaver"—tips and shortcuts that save you money.

3. "Watch Out!"—more serious cautions and warnings.

4. "Bright Idea"—general tips and shortcuts to help you find an easier or smarter way to do something.

5. "Quote"—statements from real people that are intended to be prescriptive and valuable to you.

6. "Unofficially..."—an insider's fact or anecdote.

We also recognize your need to have quick information at your fingertips, and have thus provided the following comprehensive sections at the back of the book:

1. **Glossary:** Definitions of complicated terminology and jargon.

2. **Resource Guide:** Lists of relevant agencies, associations, institutions, web sites, etc.

3. **Recommended Reading List:** Suggested titles that can help you get more in-depth information on related topics.

4. **Important Documents:** "Official" pieces of information you need to refer to, such as government forms.

5. **Important Statistics:** Facts and numbers presented at-a-glance for easy reference.

6. **Index.**

Letters, Comments, and Questions from Readers

We strive to continually improve the *Unofficial* series, and input from our readers is a valuable way for us to do that. Many of those who have used the *Unofficial Guide* travel books write to the authors to ask questions, make comments, or share their own discoveries and lessons. For lifestyle *Unofficial Guides,* we would also appreciate all such correspondence, both positive and critical, and we will make best efforts to incorporate appropriate readers' feedback and comments in revised editions of this work.

How to write to us:

Unofficial Guides
Macmillan Lifestyle Guides
Macmillan Publishing
1633 Broadway
New York, NY 10019

Attention: Reader's Comments

The *Unofficial Guide* Panel of Experts

The Unofficial editorial team recognizes that you've purchased this book with the expectation of getting the most authoritative, carefully inspected information currently available. Toward that end, on each and every title in this series, we have selected a minimum of two "official" experts comprising the "Unofficial Panel" who painstakingly review the manuscripts to ensure: factual accuracy of all data, inclusion of the most up-to-date and relevant information; and that, from an insider's perspective, the authors have armed you with all the necessary facts you need—but the institutions don't want you to know.

For *The Unofficial Guide to Overcoming Infertility*, we are proud to introduce the following panel of experts:

Sami David, M.D. Dr. David is an Assistant Clinical Professor of Obstetrics and Gynecology at the Mt. Sinai School of Medicine in New York City. A graduate of the Columbia University School of Medicine, he completed his fellowship in Reproductive Endocrinology at the

University of Pennsylvania, and has co-authored articles in medical journals on endometriosis, recurrent pregnancy loss and sperm antibodies. Dr. David has a private infertility practice in New York City where, in addition to the medical and surgical treatment of infertility in women of all ages, he specializes in the treatment of infertility in women over 39, and in recurrent pregnancy loss. He is a member of the American Society of Reproductive Medicine, the American Society of Reproductive Immunology, and is on the medical advisory board of RESOLVE NYC.

Harris Nagler, M.D. Dr. Nagler is Chariman of the Department of Urology at Beth Isreal Medicine Center and a Professor of Urology at Albert Einstein College of Medicine of Yeshiva University in New York City. Dr. Nagler is a nationally-recognized expert on the evaluation and treatment of male-factor infertility, and has published extensively on the subject in medical journals. He is a member of the American Urological Association and the American Society of Reproductive medicine. He is also a member and past president of the Society of Reproductive Surgeons and is on the medical advisory board of RESOLVE NYC. He lectures frequently at their national and local meetings, and post-graduate courses. Dr. Nagler has a faculty practice in general urology and male infertility at the Beth Israel Medical Center in New York City.

Introduction

I f you are dealing with the problem of infertility, the first and most important thing to keep in mind is this: You are not alone. According to the National Survey of Family Growth (NSFG), one of the most reliable sources of nationally representative data on the use of infertility services, of the 60.2 million women of reproductive age in 1995, 15 percent, or 9.3 million, had used some kind of infertility service. That means either they sought medical advise, underwent testing, received drugs, or underwent surgery or other treatments. That was up from the 12 percent, or 6.8 million women, in 1988.

About 2 percent of women of reproductive age (that's about 1.2 million women) had an infertility visit in the past year. Another 13 percent had received infertility services at some time in their lives prior to that year.

Help is Available

Infertility, in other words, is a much more common problem than you might have thought. But take heart. According to an article authored by assisted reproductive technology pioneer Dr. Howard Jones, the National Center for Health Statistics in 1988 reported that while 8.4 percent of women aged 15 to 44 years had an impaired ability to have children, about half of those who sought help eventually conceived. And, that was before the most recent advances in assisted reproductive technology.

While many people associate infertility treatment with these advanced technologies, the fact is that only 3 percent of all infertile couples who enter treatment go on to try in vitro fertilization. This implies that many other effective forms of treatment are available for both men and women. Fertility drugs can help women who do not produce eggs. Semen analyses can detect infections or other problems which are often relatively simple to correct.

And that's the good news of this book: With the proper medical diagnosis and treatment, more than half of all infertile couples will conceive their own biological children. Other infertile couples may be able to conceive with the aid of donor sperm or donor eggs.

Population Trends and Their Impact on Infertility Care

The statistics on infertility may seem daunting, but they are in part a reflection of certain demographic realities in today's society. For one thing, they reflect the large numbers of baby boomers who have delayed marriage and child bearing until a time when their reproductive ability is diminished. Widely available contraceptives have permitted them to schedule reproduction, and a trend toward marrying later in life, not to mention the increased incidence of second marriages—and the desire to start a second family—have contributed to the increase in demand for infertility care.

You'll note that this *Unofficial Guide* places particular emphasis on age and its relation to fertility and successful treatment. Science is accumulating mountains of evidence on how advancing age impairs not only fertility, but also the chances of successful treatment. It's vitally important that you realize that if you're a woman over the age of 35 and are even *thinking* that you may want to conceive some day, there is no time to waste. You should be preparing yourself to maximize your chances of conceiving. Unlike men in whom fertility doesn't appear to decline until after age 55, conception and complications during pregnancy are more common the older a woman is.

Over the past decade, three major changes in the field of infertility care have occurred:

1. Older women—even over age 55—are giving birth thanks to donor eggs.

2. Infertile men, for whom very little once could be offered beyond surgical correction for very specific and usually rare problems, are now able to father children despite having extremely low sperm counts thanks to new sperm retrieval methods and intracytoplasmic sperm inseminations (ICSI).

3. The growth and increased accessibility of the Internet.

The Impact of the Internet

This last development has had a profound impact on the field of infertility. The Internet can be a source of both good and bad information. Many reputable organizations, such as the RESOLVE and the American Society of Reproductive Medicine, have web sites that will provide up-to-date accurate guidelines. And this broadbased accessibility of information is a very good thing. (But do be wary when looking at other web sites or chat rooms: Keep in mind that the information isn't always from bona fide and unbiased groups.) You can learn a lot from reading other people's stories. For example, in the course of writing this book we came across an article printed on the Internet by a woman who had been a surrogate three times. Her last surrogacy arrangement did not go well. Whether her story was true or not doesn't really matter. It raised important ethical, legal, and social questions.

Reading this *Unofficial Guide* can help you avoid unnecessary, unsuccessful, or unproved treatments; maximize your chances of a successful pregnancy; teach you how to be an informed patient so that you can make decisions that are right for you; give you hints on surviving the emotional crisis of infertility and getting through some of the physical discomforts associated with some infertility tests and procedures; and outline the pros and cons of third-party reproduction. It is designed to give you the scoop on traditional and non-traditional approaches to infertility and to help you maximize your chances of getting reimbursed from your insurance company.

Our Message to You

This book arose out of the collaboration among three authors with very different, but overlapping professional backgrounds: Dr. Joan Liebmann-Smith is a medical sociologist; Jacqueline Nardi Egan, a medical writer and editor; and Dr. John Stangel, a board-certified reproductive endocrinologist. We are united by a common interest in infertility and a commitment to help couples with fertility problems.

The synergy that brought the three of us together had its beginnings when one of us, Joan, was struggling with her own infertility problems. This was back in the early 1980s, when the subject was still very new. Louise Brown, the world's first "test-tube baby" was a still an infant. Magazines were only beginning to publish stories about the subject, and there were just a handful of books available to the lay reader. Joan found one of those books to be extremely helpful. It was *The Essential Guide for Infertile Couples*, by John Stangel, MD. When Joan later became co-president of the New York chapter of RESOLVE, a national organization for infertile couples, she invited John to be a keynote speaker at their first all-day infertility symposium.

While John's book focused mostly on the medical aspects of infertility, Joan recognized a need for a book that dealt with the social and emotional aspects of the problem. Out of that recognition, Joan produced her own book, *In Pursuit of Pregnancy*, in 1987. By that time, the whole subject of infertility had come out of the closet in a big way. You couldn't open a woman's magazine without finding a story on infertility. In fact, Jacqueline Egan wrote one of the first articles for a major national publication on the pioneering work done in in vitro fertilization (IVF). But IVF was still a rarity and offered at only a handful of medical centers in this country. One of the largest and most successful of these programs in the US was IVF Australia (later called IVF America), and John Stangel became the medical director of their Westchester division.

In 1989, IVF Australia was looking for medical writers and Joan applied. So did Jacqueline. Both were hired and wound up "job sharing"—a concept that was almost as new as IVF at the time. Jacqueline tended to write mostly for the physicians and the other members of the infertility team while Joan primarily wrote patient newsletters and other patient education materials. Since John was the medical director, all three of us frequently collaborated.

A lot has changed in the years since we first collaborated. New, more effective hormonal treatments are helping an increasing number of infertile couples become pregnant. There are several hundred reproductive centers in the U.S. alone offering IVF and more advanced reproductive technologies. IVF is now a fairly simple outpatient procedure. Success rates have improved considerably, and are expected to continue to improve. And little Louise Brown is now over 21.

With these advances in the assisted reproductive technologies (ARTs) have come a host of both anticipated and unanticipated ethical issues. And, as a result, you can barely turn on your TV without seeing a story on infertility, the ARTs, multiple births, and multiple ethical dilemmas. Indeed, just as this *Unofficial Guide* went to press, the news of the first known surviving set of octuplets (one of whom died shortly thereafter) was released. The mother had taken infertility drugs and had lost a set of triplets just the year before.

What hasn't changed, however, is the emotional turmoil people suffering from infertility experience and the myriad of medical decisions they must make. This *Unofficial Guide* will help you and your partner navigate the complex world of infertility.

A Personal Message from John Stangel, MD

This is a "how-to" book. But, unlike most books in this category that tell you how to build an object or acquire a skill, this book will guide you through the many reproductive treatment choices to maximize your chances of having a child of your own. This may be one of the most important "how-to" books you will ever read.

If you are or believe you may be infertile you need accurate up-to-date information. This book is a complete and current source written in an easy-to-read format. Our knowledge of human reproduction has progressed so rapidly in the last few years—and even months—that even if you have read extensively in the field you will still benefit by reading this *Unofficial Guide*. This is the state of the art as of this very afternoon.

If you think you have an infertility problem you need to have a way of checking your concerns. If you find your concerns are real, what do you do? To whom do you go? What questions do you ask? What should your evaluation involve? How long should it take? Are there further tests that should be done? What are the treatment choices? What are the risks and benefits of each? How successful are they and are there alternatives? How much will all this cost? Will my insurance plan cover this? These are some of the questions that create the maze through which an infertile couple must travel.

Some people feel fearful just being in a doctor's office. Others are overcome with a paralyzing anxiety just going through the evaluation steps. These feelings may make it hard to absorb the information presented by your physician. If this describes you,

you may find that when you get home to review your discussion with your doctor and the information provided to you, you may remember nothing. This book can provide the missing information helping you to fill in the gaps. It can also help you formulate some questions for your doctor. In these ways, this book can help you use your time more efficiently and make the whole experience gentler.

The nightmare of every infertile couple is seeing a physician and being told: "I am sorry. There's nothing that can be done for you." It is the fear of hearing these words that keeps people from seeking help.

The good news is that it is rare for there to truly be no hope. For the vast majority of couples, a physician can find a way to help them achieve a successful pregnancy. And for those rare occasions when the words are, "I'm sorry. We can't help you.", remember, don't give up. The field of reproductive medicine is changing and progressing so quickly that what was not doable one moment is reality six months later and commonplace a year after. If having a child is important to you, do not give up. Pursue this goal aggressively. Find the right doctor. Find the right treatment and stay with it until it works.

This book can guide you through the maze of diagnosis and treatment and invisibly stand by your side offering information and support.

All of us who have worked on this book want you to succeed in your quest to have a child.

Trying...and Failing to Get Pregnant

PART I

GET THE SCOOP ON...
The human reproductive systems ▪ Sexual
practices that hamper conception ▪ Hormones
and fertility ▪ Conception ▪ Increasing your
chances of conceiving

Understanding Human Reproduction

If you're reading this book, you're already having some concerns that you're not getting pregnant as quickly as planned. Maybe you suspect that you or your partner has a fertility problem because you have never gotten pregnant, despite only sporadic contraceptive use. Or perhaps you have some medical condition that you're concerned may have affected your fertility. Or perhaps, like most people, you thought that when you decided it was the right time to get pregnant, it would just *happen*. After all, most us spend years or even decades trying very hard *not* to get pregnant—the assumption being that we're very fertile indeed.

A refresher course on conception, or back to the basics

Contrary to what you might think, most couples do not conceive the minute they start trying. In fact, an average, healthy, young couple having regular sexual relations has only a 20 percent chance of

3

"
The first
recorded infertile
woman was
Rachel, who
cried out to her
husband, Jacob,
'Give me children
or I die!'
—Genesis 30:1
"

conceiving each month, or about five to six months to conceive their first child.

Although having sex at the right time of month is a prerequisite for getting pregnant, there's a lot more required for conception to occur.

You may think you learned everything there is to know about making a baby from those late night chats with your high-school girlfriends or from your locker room buddies. If you're like most of us, you learned more myth than reality—and probably more about how *not* to get pregnant than about getting pregnant. If, like most of us, you've forgotten what you learned in high-school biology class or just didn't pay much attention, it's a good idea to think about what it really takes to conceive. Conception is a multiple-step, multi-faceted process. At any point during the process, one or more elements may not be working up to par or at all. By understanding these steps, you'll better understand:

- What can go wrong.

- Why certain diagnostic tests are performed.

- Why these tests are done at specific times during your menstrual cycle.

- Why certain medical treatments are also done at specific times of the month.

After reading this chapter you may not qualify for a medical degree, but you'll certainly be able to talk more confidently and comfortably with your doctor. Ultimately, this can save you lots of confusion, anxiety, time, and, perhaps, even money.

For conception to occur, three key factors must be in place:

- A well-functioning female reproductive system

- A well-functioning male reproductive system, and

- Effective sexual practices

The female reproductive system

Visualized from the lower portion of the female body, the main parts of a woman's reproductive system are the *vagina* (the lowermost segment), *cervix, uterus, Fallopian tubes,* and *ovaries* (the uppermost segment). These highly specialized structures have some common features:

- Some structures—such as the vagina and cervix—produce mucus, a substance that facilitates different steps during conception.

- Some—such as the uterus and Fallopian tubes—contract or undulate rhythmically, serving to move cells and tissues along the reproductive tract.

- Others—such as the ovaries and the endometrium—function through regulation by minute amounts of hormones released in specific amounts and at specific times during a woman's menstrual cycle.

Vagina

This lower structure of the female reproductive system is a long, tube-like vault. The vaginal membranes secrete a mucus that keeps the vaginal tissue soft and slippery, facilitating intercourse.

Cervix

At the end of the vagina is a small, circular area, called the cervix, which leads into the uterus, or womb. The cervix has several purposes:

Unofficially...
More than 4,000 years ago, the Egyptians were testing for pregnancy. A woman coated her shoulders, breasts, and arms with grease before going to sleep. If her skin turned "green and moist" she would most surely have a normal pregnancy.

Note! ➡
The female reproductive system.
On entering the female reproductive system, sperm follow the direction of the arrows shown in the figure.

Uterus

Fertilization usually occurs here

Ovary

Cervix

Fallopian tube

Sperm

Vagina

Timesaver
If you're in your late thirties or older, make an appointment with a fertility specialist right away (see Chapter 2). If there's a long wait list, see another recommended doctor in the meantime to start diagnostic testing. Time is truly critical!

- It helps protect the uterus and other reproductive organs against invasion by bacteria, fungi, and viruses.

- During menstruation, the endometrial lining of the uterus is shed and expelled through the cervix.

- It's through the cervix that sperm enter the uterus as they try to swim their way up to the Fallopian tubes.

- During childbirth, the cervix dilates to allow the fetus to pass through its uppermost portion, the birth canal.

The cervix also produces mucus, which, as you will learn more about later, changes consistency throughout the menstrual cycle. During most of the cycle, when a woman's not fertile, a small amount of very thick cervical mucus is present. This consistency tends to trap sperm and to block them from entering the uterus easily. But that's okay. No eggs are yet available to be fertilized anyway. In contrast, cervical mucus becomes watery and abundant during ovulation. This helps sperm swim more easily through it and up into the uterus and Fallopian tubes, on their journey to a mature egg.

Uterus

Located within the protection of the woman's pelvis, the uterus is thick-walled and muscular. It resembles an inverted sack. It is here that a fertilized egg normally implants itself in the uterine lining, is nourished, and matures for nine months until labor and delivery. During labor, the uterus contracts rhythmically and powerfully to move the fetus out of the womb into the birth canal and out through the dilated cervix and vagina. During menstruation, the uterus also contracts, though less violently, to expel the unfertilized egg and shed endometrial tissue.

The position of the uterus is described by the direction in which it leans inside the pelvis. In 80 percent of women, the uterus leans in a forward direction—this is called an *"anteverted" uterus.* If the uterus leans forward but bends in upon itself, it is called "antiflexed." Sometimes a woman is told she has *tipped uterus.* This merely means that her uterus tends to tilt backward toward her spine. A tipped uterus is also known as a *retroverted* uterus. When it is tipped backward but bends in upon itself, it's called retroflexed. It's not unusual to have a tipped uterus, and it doesn't necessarily mean that you can't conceive as some old-wives' tale suggest.

The walls of the uterus are lined with tissue called the *endometrium,* which responds to hormone changes throughout the menstrual cycle. It is the endometrium that sheds and sloughs off during menstruation.

Watch Out!
Don't totally depend on temperature charts, cervical mucus tests, and ovulation kits to dictate when to have sex. If there are no sperm to meet up with a newly released egg, you can't get pregnant.

Fallopian tubes

On each side of the uterus is a long, muscular structure, called a Fallopian tube or oviduct, which serves as a conduit for the passage of eggs to the uterus. Each part of the Fallopian tube is lined with cells covered with microscopic hairlike projections— called cilia—which move in a wave-like manner to help guide the eggs through the tubes. The ends of the Fallopian tubes are delicate, funnel-shaped structures, called *fimbria*, that catch the eggs as they are expelled from the ovaries.

The Fallopian tube lining itself produces a nutritive medium to nourish the eggs. Both the contractions of the Fallopian wall and the beating of the cilia move a fertilized egg to the uterus for implantation.

Ovaries

Perhaps the best known structures in the female reproductive system are the ovaries. These olive-sized and -shaped structures, found just beneath the Fallopian tubes and to each side of the uterus, contain eggs, each called an *ovum*. Every egg is actually housed in a bubble-like structure called a follicle. At birth, a woman has as many eggs as she will ever have in her lifetime. Each month, several are selected for possible maturation and release from the follicles.

If an ovary is missing or has been removed for a medical reason, the other takes over the monthly menstrual cycle functions. Ovulation does not alternate between ovaries, but is a random event. Some women do, however, have a dominant ovary and will ovulate from that one more than the other.

The male reproductive system

Unlike the female reproductive system, the male reproductive system has both external and internal parts. The major parts on the outside are the *testes, scrotum, epididymis,* and *penis;* on the inside are the *seminal vesicles, vas deferens,* and *prostate.* And, unlike the female's eggs that stay secure in the inner sanctum of the upper reproductive organs, the male's sperm journeys from parts in the external organs, into the internal organs, and finally out an external organ.

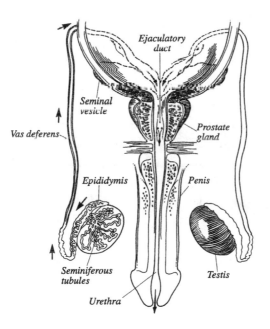

← Note!
The male reproductive system. During ejaculation, sperm follow the direction indicated by arrows in the diagram.

The testes or testicles

The *testes* are the main male sex glands. These sperm- and testosterone-producing factories are housed in a sac, called the *scrotum*, which lies below and slightly to either side of the penis. The testes contain hundreds of tightly coiled microscopic tubules called *seminiferous tubules*. It is here that sperm are produced, though they are not yet able to fertilize an egg.

Epididymis

After production in the testes, sperm leave the testicles bathed in testicular fluid and enter the epididymis. The epididymis is a 15-foot long, tightly coiled cluster of microscopic tubes attached to a testicle. Here the sperm stay about two weeks during which time they develop the ability to swim.

Vas deferens

Once mature, sperm are propelled by contractions to the end of the epididymis near an internal structure called the *vas deferens*. The vas deferens is also a tubal structure. It connects the epididymis with two other male sex glands, the *seminal vesicles* and the *prostate*. Both glands produce semen, which mixes with the sperm. Sperm and seminal fluid are stored in the vas deferens, awaiting their entrance to the urethra and out to the penis during orgasm and ejaculation.

Penis

It is through the urethra, which runs the length of the penis, that semen-containing sperm are ejaculated during orgasm. It is here that the sperm are posed for a tumultuous ride through the vas deferens at the time of orgasm and ejaculation.

Sperm

Sperm formation and maturation take about seventy two days. The chance of conception is diminished considerably if a man doesn't have millions of normally shaped, fast-moving sperm that can travel in a relatively straight line up the vagina, through the cervix, into the uterine cavity, and finally into the Fallopian tube and welcoming arms of a mature ovum.

Although only a single sperm is needed to fertilize an egg, millions are normally released with each ejaculation. Such large numbers are released to assure that a high percentage of normal, fast-moving sperm that are able to swim up to the Fallopian tube are present. After all, an egg can only be fertilized twenty-four to forty-eight hours around ovulation (some say only twelve to twenty-four hours). Having so many sperm available for whenever an egg moves down the Fallopian tube will help increase the likelihood of their meeting. Sperm are actually carried through the Fallopian tubes by contraction of the tube muscles and the beating of the tubal cilia, as well as the movement of the sperm themselves. Recent medical advances have helped men with low, or even very low, sperm counts to produce children.

Female hormones—the language of her reproductive cycle

Menstruation, fertility, conception, and, if successful, labor, are orchestrated elegantly by the rise and fall of hormone levels.

The human body, whether male or female, houses many different glands that produce a wide variety of hormones. Traveling through the bloodstream to special target tissues, hormones act as

Watch Out! Because high temperatures can kill sperm, the man should avoid hot tubs, saunas, and steam rooms— particularly prior to sexual intercourse.

chemical messengers to regulate the myriad bodily functions, from blood pressure control and thyroid function to urine output, and, of course, fertility.

If you aren't already, you should become knowledgeable about the different female and male hormones. Your doctor:

- Will measure hormone levels to help diagnose a cause of infertility

- May prescribe hormones to correct imbalances and improve the chance of conception

- May monitor hormone levels to pinpoint the best times for different procedures and treatments

In this section we will talk about the female sex hormones and their function during the menstrual cycle and conception.

Note! ➡
During a normal menstrual cycle, the balance of four reproductive hormones shifts, reflecting changes in the body's body temperature.

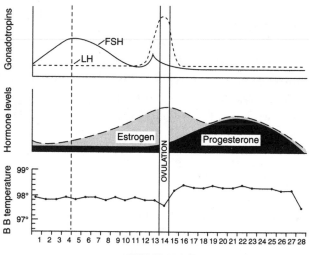

DAY OF CYCLE

GnRH

The menstrual cycle begins as signals are sent from the *hypothalamus,* a specialized area just above the *pituitary gland* at the base of the brain. Every 60 to 90 minutes, the hypothalamus pumps out a hormone called *gonadotropin-releasing hormone (GnRH)* for about one minute. GnRH stimulates the pituitary glands above it to release two more hormones, *follicle-stimulating hormone (FSH)* and *luteinizing hormone (LH).*

FSH and LH

Called *gonadotropin hormones* and produced by the pituitary, FSH is critical during the first half of the menstrual cycle, called the *follicular phase* and LH is critical during the second half, called the *luteal phase.*

The first day of a woman's menstrual period signals Day 1 of a new menstrual cycle. On that day, the pituitary releases FSH, which signals the ovaries to increase production of the major female hormone *estrogen.* Under the influence of estrogen, the uterine lining, or endometrium, enters a proliferative phase, that is, it grows and thickens, in preparation for implantation by the fertilized egg.

As its name implies, FSH causes several follicles—which house the eggs—in the ovaries to develop and ripen. By Day 7, one of the follicles begins to grow rapidly. The other lag behind are are eventually absorbed by the body.

By Day 14, of an ideal 28-day cycle, LH begins to take over. There is a sudden, dramatic rise in LH levels, called the *LH surge,* which culminates in *ovulation.* During the surge, LH helps stimulate several important follicular functions. Like every cell in the human body, the egg cell has 46 chromosomes—

Unofficially...
Many animals are more efficient at conception than humans. Pigs ejaculate almost a pint of semen. To ensure that none leaks out, the male pig's penis actually has grooves that link up with grooves in the female pig's cervix.

Timesaver
Start compiling
medical records
from your doc-
tors now. Include
OB-GYNs, urolo-
gists, and any
other specialists
you've seen.

strands of genetic material. The LH surge prepares the egg cell to expel half of its chromosomes. (Sperm, the male reproductive cells, also each has forty-six chromosomes to start. They, too, must shed half their chromosomes before meeting up with a mature egg. In this way the fertilized egg will have a full complement of chromosomes—half from the egg and half from the sperm.)

LH also helps ripen the follicle further, causing it to rupture and release a mature egg. The ovum, or egg, is expelled from the follicle on the ovary, grabbed by the fimbria at the end of the Fallopian tube, and journeys down the narrow Fallopian tube on the road to possible fertilization.

Progesterone

LH then signals the remnant of the newly ovulated follicle that has just released an egg to become a sort of endocrine gland, the *corpus luteum*. LH tells the corpus luteum to produce another major female sex hormone, *progesterone*. Like estrogen, progesterone, targets the uterine tissue lining.

When it reaches the uterus, progesterone prompts the lining to undergo a change that enables it to support and nourish a newly fertilized egg. This preparation of the uterine lining takes approximately five days, the same time it takes for a fertilized egg to reach the cavity of the uterus.

Estrogen

Estrogen is the major female sex hormone and is responsible for sex characteristics such as skin texture, hair distribution, and body contour. During the first half of the menstrual cycle, that is, the half prior to ovulation, this ovarian hormone stimulates the endometrium (uterine wall) to become lushly supplied with blood. In the second half of the cycle following ovulation, progesterone is produced. This hormone, too, acts on the endometrium, increasing the growth of secretory cells, which are needed for a new life to grow in the uterus. When progesterone is produced, it also acts on the endometrium, increasing the growth of secretory cells, which are needed for a new life to grow in the uterus.

In other words, estrogen grows the uterine lining. Progesterone makes it soft and spongy to support the life of an embryo to latch onto the endometrium. Estrogen also increases the amount and changes the consistency of cervical mucus. At approximately Day 14 of the menstrual cycle, estrogen causes cervical mucus production to increase and the mucus to become thinner.

If pregnancy does not occur, the corpus luteum degenerates and progesterone production ceases after fourteen days. Estrogen production tapers off during the second or luteal phase of the menstrual cycle. Deprived of hormonal support, the top layer of the endometrium begins to pull away from the uterine wall. No longer able to maintain this state of anticipation or preparation for a fertilized egg, the uterine lining crumbles and sloughs off. Rhythmic uterine contractions expel the built-up blood, the extra growth of the uterine lining, and the disintegrated egg. This is the menstrual discharge that flows through the cervix into the vagina over a three-to-five-day period marking the end of one reproductive cycle and the beginning of another.

HCG

If pregnancy occurs and the fertilized egg starts implanting in the uterine wall, the early pregnancy begins to produce *human chorionic gonadotropin (HCG)*. HCG is usually produced only when a

Unofficially...
Because a child conceived by intoxicated parents was thought to be unhealthy, the ancient cities of Carthage and Sparta prohibited newlyweds from drinking alcoholic beverages.

fertilized egg reaches the implantation stage. Sometimes called the "pregnancy hormone," HCG is necessary to support a pregnancy. In fact, it's the HCG that "switches off" the menstrual cycle and ensures that no more eggs are produced during pregnancy.

The male hormones: the language of his reproductive cycle

Like its female counterpart, the male reproductive system falls under the influence of several hormones, generally called androgens. Produced in the testes, testosterone is the primary male sex hormone. Testosterone is responsible for the characteristics of the male body, including skin texture, hair distribution, voice quality, etc.

Unofficially...
Interestingly, both men and women have many reproductive hormones in common. Women produce testosterone, and men produce estrogen. Both also produce FSH and LH.

Making love...and babies

And, finally, something that you can actively participate in and have fun while you're at it—sex. There are a great many myths perpetrated about "how to do it right" so that you increase your chances to conceive. With the exception of only a few "don'ts," you've probably been doing it just fine. Besides, if you think you have a fertility problem or you've been diagnosed with one, you'll likely be asked to engage in sexual intercourse at times when the mood doesn't necessarily strike you. There's no reason to add to the burden of making sure your technique is flawless, too. These are not the "Sexual Olympics" and getting a "Perfect 10" isn't going to assure conception.

Here are two common notions about sexual practices that both couples and physicians sometimes put a great deal of stock into. But, in fact, they would be hard to prove or disprove:

■ **The position you use matters.** Many people assume that if the female partner is on top during sexual intercourse, sperm will leak out of the vagina, reducing the chances for conception. Somehow, the sperm seem to make it to where they need to be whether the couple engages in the missionary position or not. The force of the ejaculation, whether the man is on top or not, is enough to propel sperm into the cervical mucus. It's only the sperm that get into the cervical mucus that will pass through the cervix and enter the uterus. Whatever sperm don't reach the cervical mucus then will probably be rendered useless in the vaginal environment anyway. So, use the position that's most comfortable for you. It's having sexual intercourse that's important.

■ **Stay in bed for twenty to thirty minutes after intercourse.** This is a corollary to the "get-into-the-right-position" belief. Some women have been told that rushing out of bed will cause millions of sperm to flow out of the vagina. But while there doesn't appear to be any medical justification for this advice, many women feel better staying put for a few minutes. Because trying to conceive can put enormous strains on a couple, languishing in bed a bit in the afterglow of the moment may be soothing. Enjoy the quite time together.

Here are a few things, however, that *are* important:

■ **You have to do it to get pregnant.** Not having vaginal intercourse because of discomfort when the penis enters the vagina (dyspareunia), impotence, or lack of interest makes conceiving

Bright Idea
Under some circumstances, gravity might increase your odds of conceiving. If ejaculate volume is small, sperm count low, and semen viscous, the missionary position may be your best bet.

difficult, if not, impossible. Engaging in only anal or oral intercourse when the woman is ovulating will miss a prime opportunity for conception, too.

■ If possible, don't use vaginal lubricants. Certainly, don't use ones that contain spermicides—as their name says, they kill sperm. It's a good idea to read the labels or ask your doctor or pharmacist about their contents. Even lubricants without spermicides can hamper sperm mobility. Body oils and creams can trap sperm, too. If you must use a lubricant, choose only water-soluble ones. Of course, the best lubricants are the vaginal secretions themselves. Even saliva can harm sperm.

■ Optimize your fertile time. In essence, you should time sexual intercourse to maximize your most fertile time. If you're trying to get pregnant, it's a good idea to have sex at every other day around the time you ovulate. That means on Day 10, 12, 14, and 16 of an ideal 28-day menstrual cycle. The reason: sperm are viable for about 48 hours. This pattern helps assure that enough sperm are present whenever the woman ovulates and it gives the male partner some time to build up a good sperm supply for the next ejaculation. Having sex every other day beginning on Day 10 will keep sufficient sperm around when an egg shows up.

Here's a tip for knowing when to have sex during your most fertile time: Determine the length of your cycle. (Remember, the first day of your menstrual period is the first day of your cycle.) Subtract 14 days. The interval that includes that cycle day and the four days before

Bright Idea
Here's a reason to have sex more often: Studies have shown that couples who have sex less than once a week are unlikely to conceive within the first six months of trying.

and the two days after is the optimal time. If there's no known problem with the sperm, every day to every other day, as the two of you desire, would be the best rule. The LH kit can tighten this up even more. Have sex one day prior to the darkest color test result to one day after the darkest color.

The journey towards conception

When the male ejaculates during intercourse, as many as one hundred million sperm are released into the vagina. Despite this enormous, mobile army, only a few hundred or thousand sperm reach the Fallopian tube where the egg or eggs are. The other hundreds of thousands are lost, falling prey to a very hostile environment. Here are some of the problems sperm may encounter once in the vagina:

- Many sperm are killed by the vaginal environment.

- Cervical mucus may be too thick to allow the sperm to penetrate it and enter the uterus.

- Sperm cell movement may be so poor that too few can survive. In rare cases, the cervical mucus may contain antibodies that can incapacitate sperm. It's unclear, however, how significant, if any, these antibodies are in preventing pregnancy or causing infertility.

- Once out of the vagina, sperm movement may be hampered by structural damage in the uterus or tubes, making it mechanically difficult for sperm to reach an egg.

- Of course, if too few sperm are ejaculated, or if their quality is poor, not enough sperm may be present to make the journey.

Moneysaver
At mid-cycle, try using Robitussin or any other over-the-counter cough syrup that contains expectorants. Expectorants can improve the quality of your cervical mucus at a fraction of the cost of fertility drugs. But make certain the expectorant doesn't contain an antihistamine that can dry out the mucus, making matters worse. A good rule: If it drys out your nose, it will dry out your vagina.

Of those sperm that reach the cervical canal, half enter the wrong Fallopian tube in search of an absent egg. Of those that enter the correct Fallopian tube, many are lost in the maze of the tube's folds. During this journey, the remaining sperm will undergo a process called *capacitation*, which gives them the capacity to penetrate and fertilize an egg.

From egg to embryo: in eight sometimes not-so-easy steps

Pregnancy is not an instantaneous event. It's a sequence of physiological milestones that take place over several days.

1. **Ovulation**. This is the first, but sometimes, most difficult step in the path to pregnancy. Mid-cycle each month, a mature egg, or ovum, is released from its follicle on the ovary surface.

2. **Fertilization**. When a single sperm penetrates the dense outer coat surrounding the ovum, called the *zona pellucida*. This coat makes the ovum impervious to other sperm and fertilization occurs. The single cell that results from this fertilization is called the *zygote*.

3. **Cleavage**. Beginning a few hours after fertilization, the zygote begins its long, dramatic growth—starting with a single cell, dividing, and redividing. First, two cells are formed, then four, then eight—the number of cells doubling with each division.

4. As the zygote continues to divide, it travels down the Fallopian tube into the uterus. Although the number of cells increases with each division, the size of the cells becomes smaller. If the overall size of the zygote increased, it would become too large to travel down the narrow passageways of the Fallopian tube into the uterus.

Watch Out!
It's probably not a good idea to douche just before or after intercourse. Check the labels on douches; they may contain spermicides.

5. As we said earlier, the fertilized egg enters the uterus—powered by the muscular contractions of the Fallopian tube and guided by the minute, fringe-like projections on the tube's surface. The rapidly dividing zygote lies here for two to three days, growing and differentiating into cells that are destined to perform various functions.

6. **Blastocyst**. On Day 7 after fertilization, the fertilized egg loses its protective coating. This new hollow sphere of cells floating freely in the uterine cavity is called a *blastocyst*. The blastocyst must now attach, or implant, itself in the uterine wall.

7. **Trophoblast**. Now totaling about 100 cells, the blastocyst nestles against the uterine wall and prepares to attach itself. At this stage the blastocyst has two distinct portions—an inner cell mass and an outer wall of flattened cells called the *trophoblast*. (This trophoblast becomes a hormone-producing organism, secreting *human chorionic gonadotropin (HCG)*.

8. **Implantation**. During implantation, the trophoblastic cells penetrate the uterine wall, embedding themselves into the endometrium. The blastocyst is firmly attached, or implanted, by Day 12 after fertilization.

A blastocyst sometimes becomes implanted inside the Fallopian tube or somewhere other than inside the uterine cavity. This is called an *ectopic pregnancy*. Such pregnancies are life-threatening and are usually terminated either surgically or with the use of medications.

The trophoblast is designed to become the nutritional organ of the embryo; the inner cell mass will become the embryo itself. The point where they meet becomes the umbilical cord.

During implantation, the trophoblast grows finger-like projections into the surrounding maternal tissue. They radiate out like porcupine quills, and are call *villi*. The villi pierce the lush blood channels in the endometrium, which allows the villi to be microscopically bathed in nourishing blood. These villous lakes are the start of a new organ growing between the embryo and the mother. Called a *chorion*, it permits material circulation to sustain and nourish the embryo. Part of the chorion will form the placenta, which becomes a hormone-producing organ that supports the pregnancy.

When everything goes right

Although you now probably know more about reproduction than most beginning medical students, the following will help you understand the process of conception in a nutshell:

- The woman must ovulate a healthy, ripe, fertilizable egg.
- Fallopian tubes must be unobstructed in order to receive the egg.
- The couple must have sexual intercourse prior to or at the time of ovulation.
- The man must ejaculate millions of healthy, viable sperm deep into the woman's vagina.
- Many sperm must travel through the cervix into the uterus and finally into the open Fallopian tubes.
- The egg must be fertilized in the Fallopian tube and then travel back into the uterus.

- The fertilized egg must implant itself in a hormonally primed, normally shaped uterus, and grow into a healthy embryo.

You can see where there is a lot of room for error, and why it takes so long for many couples, both fertile and infertile, to conceive.

When everything seems to be going wrong

Don't panic. You may or may not have a fertility problem. Even if you do, infertility treatments have become so advanced that your chances for conceiving are better than ever. But before you start running off to fertility specialists, there is a lot you can do in preparation, or while you're waiting for that first appointment.

Take control of the situation

Whether or not you're certain you have a fertility problem, there are some basic steps you should take before you start infertility treatment.

- Get a physical examination. Both partners should be in good physical condition before starting a family. But since the woman is the one who becomes pregnant and gives birth, she especially needs to be healthy. She also needs to be aware of any conditions she might have than can hinder her chances of conceiving. A routine physical exam might turn up some condition that can interfere with your fertility such as diabetes, thyroid disorders, sexually transmitted diseases or even being too under- or overweight. An early diagnosis and treatment can save you considerable costs, both financial and emotional, of infertility treatment. If anything is found, go to a fertility specialist sooner, rather than later.

- If you haven't gotten pregnant within six months, the male partner should go for a semen analysis. Although this will ultimately have to be done and even repeated several times, doing it early can save time and even needless testing and treatment. Many women have gone through years of expensive, invasive infertility treatments only later to discover that their husbands have low sperm counts.

Determine if and when you're ovulating

"

When my doctor told me to keep track of my temperature every morning, I wasn't sure what she meant. She told me I could take it orally, rectally, or vaginally, even at night, as long as I was consistent.
—Sally, a twenty-nine-year-old teacher

"

Normal conception can't occur without ovulation. Luckily, there are some easy, fairly accurate, noninvasive ways of determining whether or not you ovulate, and even pinpointing the time of ovulation. In addition, these simple methods can help determine whether or not you ovulate regularly, and whether or not your cycles are abnormally long or short. (In Chapter 2, we will go into more detail about how to interpret ovulation tests.)

- Keep a temperature chart for three to four months. This is commonly referred to as charting your basal body temperature (BBT). It involves taking your oral temperature each morning before you get out of bed or each evening just before bedtime. The important thing is to be consistent and to accurately record the results on a chart. You should also indicate the days you menstruate and the days—or nights—when you have intercourse. This will not only help you pinpoint ovulation, but will give you some idea of whether or not you are, in fact, ovulating.

- Monitor your body for signs of ovulation. Many women feel a twinge, pain or discomfort in or around the ovaries when they ovulate. This sensation is called *"mittleschmertz."*

- Check your cervical mucus. The quality and quantity of cervical mucus changes throughout the menstrual cycle. Sperm do not live in sticky, opaque mucus, but survive very nicely in moist, stretchy mucus. As you get closer to ovulation, your cervical mucus will become thinner, clearer, and more stretchable. When the mucus can be stretched an inch or more without breaking, sperm penetration is most likely to occur. This characteristic of cervical mucus is called *spinnbarkheit.* In order to check the quality of your cervical mucus, you insert your finger into your vagina and get a small sample of mucus on your finger from around your cervix. Then try to stretch the mucus between your finger and thumb.

- Buy an ovulation prediction kit. By testing your urine each day and charting the results, you can help determine whether or not you ovulate and the optimal time to have sex. They cost between $15 and $60. Although you have to buy a new kit each month, they are more accurate than BBT charting.

Other ways of taking control of your fertility

By reading this book, you've taken a major step toward being in control of your fertility. But don't stop here. It's important for you to become an expert on infertility. After all, you want to do everything you can to become pregnant. Educating yourself about the process is essential.

Moneysaver
Shop around for ovulation kits at discount pharmacies, or order from mail order catalogues. The prices can vary from $15 to $60.

Timesaver
If you see from your BBT charts and the ovulation kits that you have a regular cycle, you can probably free yourself of the daily ritual of temperature taking.

■ Read everything you can about infertility. Go to bookstores, public libraries, and medical libraries if you have access. Don't be intimidated by the medical books or terms. While you won't necessarily understand everything you read, they can be helpful, especially as you progress through diagnosis and treatment.

■ Use the internet. The internet provides a wealth of information on infertility, as well as the opportunity to talk to others about infertility and maintain your anonymity if you'd like. Get on infertility web sites and into infertility chat rooms. We've listed many web sites and other sources of information in the appendix. But read everything with a critical eye. Not all information on the internet is accurate.

■ Join RESOLVE, a national organization for infertile couples that has 55 chapters in 47 cities across the nation. RESOLVE provides information on all aspects of infertility, puts out newsletters, offers lists of qualified fertility specialists, and provides emotional support. If there isn't a chapter of RESOLVE in your community, try to find another support group.

Just the facts

■ Make sure you and your partner are healthy.

■ Stop any unhealthy habits (smoking, alcohol, and caffeine use) before you try to get pregnant.

■ Become aware of your body, its hormonal rhythms and signs of ovulation.

■ Have a baseline sperm evaluation before subjecting yourselves to more invasive and expensive testing.

- Don't be hesitant to question even your simplest habits, such as sexual practices and dieting. They may be interfering with your fertility, but are the easiest to correct.

- Become informed—you've made a great start by reading this *Unofficial Guide*.

GET THE SCOOP ON...
Odds of conception as you age ▪ The effect of
disease on fertility ▪ Fertility and your lifestyle
▪ Over-the-counter and prescription drugs ▪
Common myths and misconceptions

Understanding Infertility

If you think you have a fertility problem, you may feel all alone. But you're not. In fact, infertility affects more than 6 million American women and their partners. That's about 10 percent of Americans who are of reproductive age. Some estimates put the figure as high as 20 percent! Infertility affects men and women with almost equal frequency.

It's important to remember that many different conditions can affect your ability to conceive. But it's equally important to remember that recent advances in drug therapy, microsurgery, and assisted reproductive technologies are making it possible for half to three-quarters of the couples seeking treatment to conceive.

In Chapter 1 we reviewed the female and male reproductive systems and the hormones that regulate them. In this chapter, we'll look at what factors can impair these systems and throw hormones off balance. But first, it will be helpful to define some of the terminology used when talking about infertility. You'll be seeing and hearing these terms frequently throughout this book, other resources on infertility, and, especially, when you talk to your doctor.

What is infertility?

There is a lot of confusion about the term *infertility*. Many people think that infertility means *sterility*, which is defined as the absolute inability to reproduce. While some infertile men and women are indeed sterile, involuntary sterility is a very rare condition. On the other hand, millions of American couples are diagnosed as infertile each year.

The actual definition of infertility is the inability of a couple to achieve a successful pregnancy after one year of unprotected sexual intercourse. A woman is infertile, therefore, if she cannot become pregnant or carry a pregnancy to full term after a year of trying, and a man is infertile if he cannot impregnate a woman after a year of trying. Infertile men are also commonly referred to as *subfertile*. While sterility is usually incurable, the majority of infertile couples ultimately do conceive. *Secondary infertility* is the term used to describe a man or woman who has previously had a biological child. Those who have never had children are said to have *primary infertility*.

A couple is said to have *unexplained infertility* when, after going through extensive diagnostic procedures, no cause for their inability to conceive is found. While in 84 percent of the cases a problem is found with the man, woman, or both, in the remaining 16 percent, no definitive problem with either partner is pinpointed. That's not to say that there's nothing wrong with the couple. It's just that existing diagnostic methods are not perfect.

Timesaver
If you're told—particularly in the early phases of diagnosis and treatment—that you have unexplained infertility, go to another fertility specialist for a second opinion. Another doctor may pick up on something the first one missed. And be sure your partner has another semen analysis. Sperm count can change dramatically within a few months.

Unexplained infertility is extremely frustrating for both the couple and the physician. Even though a cause for your fertility problem may not be found, there are a variety of treatments that can be used to increase your chances of getting pregnant. The good news is that in the majority of these cases, the couple becomes pregnant either spontaneously or through treatment.

What is female factor infertility? What about male factor?

In the past, it was not uncommon for the medical profession, as well as many couples, to assume that the cause of infertility was entirely due to the woman. Fortunately, more and more of society is recognizing that something may be amiss in the man, as well as the woman. Indeed, infertility can be caused by a number of factors attributable to the woman, the man, or both.

The term *female factor* is used to describe conditions or disorders in a woman that contribute to infertility; *male factor* is used to describe those conditions or disorders in a man that are the cause of an infertility problem.

Successful conception and pregnancy depends on many factors, as we saw in Chapter 1. Sometimes more than one aspect is off balance. Individually neither would impact greatly on your ability to conceive, but together they throw the odds against you. A woman who has a subtle cervical mucus problem might not have trouble conceiving if her partner has a normal sperm count. However, if her partner has a low sperm count, her chances of conceiving are greatly reduced.

> 66
> Those who are beyond the fourteenth or fifteenth year of age, not too long nor too thick, not too fat, not too flabby, not too moist or too dry, with crevices not too open nor too closed, those who menstruate regularly—these are fertile. Those who do not possess large fleshy loins and are mannish in their physique are sterile.
> —Soranus, Roman Physician, 2nd century AD
> 99

Common conditions that can affect you and/or your partner

Before looking more closely at the most common causes of infertility in women and men separately, it's a good idea to take a quick look at some conditions and situations that can affect either sex. If any of these affects you, bring it to your doctor's attention early. In some cases, there are measures you can take or treatments you can receive that will quickly improve your chances of conceiving. For others, you will save valuable time and expense in diagnosing and correcting a problem.

Age and infertility

In many cases of infertility, unexplained or otherwise, the problem turns out to be a function of age. A doctor may not find anything definitively wrong with you, but the reality is, the older you are, the harder it is to become pregnant.

There has been a dramatic rise in the numbers of couples seeking treatment for infertility. In fact, there was a 30 percent increase in the number of women being treated for infertility between 1988 and 1995. This increase is primarily due to the fact that many baby-boomers have delayed childbearing until their thirties or even fourties. In fact, 20 percent of couples now wait until they're over thirty-five to have their first child.

The longer a woman waits to try to conceive, the longer it will take her. The optimal time for a woman to conceive is between the ages of twenty-two and twenty-six. However, many women in their early twenties do not want to conceive—they may not be married, or they may be busy pursuing their education or careers, or they just may not yet feel ready to start their families.

Fertility starts declining after the age of thirty and more rapidly after thirty-five. A woman under thirty has about a 20 percent chance of conceiving each month. By the time she reaches forty, her chances of conceiving drop to only 5 percent each month.

Why is this? After age thirty, hormone levels start declining and eggs start deteriorating subtly. A woman is born with all her eggs—about 300,000. But as she approaches menopause, only a few thousand eggs—eggs that have been around for a lifetime—are left. And older eggs are not only not as fertilizable as young eggs, they're much more likely to carry chromosomal abnormalities such as Down Syndrome. But if you're older, don't despair—the majority of older women who carry a pregnancy to term give birth to healthy babies.

Fertility among men also decreases with age, although not as dramatically as for women. Older men tend to have lower levels of testosterone, and this in turn affects their sexual drive, as well as their ability to achieve and maintain an erection. Older men are also more likely to have medical conditions, such as *atherosclerosis* (hardening of the arteries) or diabetes, that can impair sexual ability.

In addition, older couples tend to have sex less often than younger couples. And the older you are, the greater the chances are that you have gotten illnesses that can interfere with your fertility, such as sexually transmitted diseases (STDs), diabetes, and thyroid disease.

Unofficially...
In the eighteenth century ectopic pregnancies were believed to be the result of extramarital affairs.

TABLE 2.1: HOW MATERNAL AGE AFFECTS PREGNANCY RATE

Age	Cumulative Pregnancy Rate	Monthly Pregnancy Rate
Under 30	74	10.5
31 to 35	61	9.1
Over 35	54	6.5

Source: E. H. Illinions, M. T. Valley, and A. M. Kaunitz, "Infertility: A Clinical Guide For The Internist." Med Clin N. Am. 1998; 82(2): 271-291.

Recurrent miscarriage

While the chance of conceiving decreases the older one gets, the chance of *miscarriage*, or *spontaneous abortion*, as it is called in the medical field, increases. Miscarriage is a relatively common occurrence. Ten to 12 percent of pregnancies in women under thirty-five years of age end in miscarriage; 18 percent of those between thirty-five and thirty-nine, and 34 percent of those between forty and forty-four, do as well. More than half the pregnant women forty-five or over miscarry.

TABLE 2.2: PERCENTAGE OF PREGNANCIES ENDING IN MISCARRIAGE, BY AGE

Age of woman at pregnancy	Percentage ending in miscarriage
Under 35 years	10 to 12
Between 35 and 39	18
Between 40 and 44	34
45 or over	>50

Source: P. R. Gindoff and R. Jewelewicz, "Reproductive Potential in the Older Woman." *Fertility and Sterility*, 1986; 46: 989.

While even one miscarriage is an emotionally traumatic experience for most couples, it is only considered a medical problem if a woman miscarries repeatedly—at least three times, or in women at high risk, like those older than age 35, twice. This is referred to as *recurrent miscarriage* or *habitual abortion*, and warrants further investigation. If you're older than 35, you should probably seek medical evaluation after two consecutive miscarriages.

The causes of miscarriage can be hormonal, genetic or chromosomal, immunological, or structural (the uterus can't hold the baby, or the cervix opens prematurely). Infections, diseases, certain drugs, chemicals and environmental toxins, caffeine, tobacco, and alcohol have also been implicated as causes of miscarriages. Some activities can also increase your chances of miscarriage. For example, while physically fit, experienced women skiers can continue their sport during early pregnancy, high-altitude skiing is ill advised. In addition, women should avoid prolonged use of hot tubs and scuba diving during pregnancy.

Although the findings are controversial, some studies have also linked the timing of sexual intercourse to miscarriage. In one study, miscarriage was highest when conception took place three days after ovulation. The chances of miscarriage were lowest in women who conceived right when they ovulated. Even lower-than-normal sperm counts have been linked to miscarriage.

Fifty to sixty percent of first trimester miscarriages are the result of genetic or chromosomal problems with the fetus. But miscarriages can occur throughout a pregnancy. Ten to fifteen percent of women with recurrent miscarriages have some sort of uterine abnormality such as a misshapen uterus. Sixteen percent of mid-trimester miscarriages are the result of cervical abnormalities. Hormonal abnormalities can cause miscarriages throughout a pregnancy. Immunological factors are also being recognized as an important cause of miscarriages,

66

Shortly before moving to this country, I suffered my second miscarriage. I was very depressed. I thought it was just Nature's way. Because my parents had died when I was very young, having a family was important to me. Then I saw a TV show about new treatments of miscarriage. I called the doctor immediately and he referred me to someone nearby.
—Lisa, mother of a healthy toddler.

99

Watch Out!
Nurses mixing chemotherapeutic agents have an almost two-fold risk of miscarriage, according to the American College of Obetetricians and Gyne-cologists.

particularly those that appear to have no other explanation.

Sexually transmitted diseases

Each year, more than 12 million cases of *sexually transmitted diseases* (*STDs*) are diagnosed in this country. STDs are a leading cause of infertility for several reasons. First, if left unrecognized and untreated, they can travel from the lower sexual organs to the upper reproductive tracts. Second, it's easy for them to go unnoticed because the most common STDs can be symptomless or may produce only vague symptoms.

Pelvic inflammatory disease

Some STDs place women at risk for *pelvic inflammatory disease* (*PID*), a widespread infection of the reproductive tract with potentially devastating results. PID is caused by the spread of organisms from the vagina and cervix to the upper reproductive tract. It is often, but not always, caused by the bacteria responsible for STDs. In fact, the dramatic rise in the incidence of PID in the last thirty years correlates strongly with the prevalence of STDs. It can be life-threatening, or it can be asymptomatic— that is, you don't even know you have it.

In the short term, PID can cause pain and discomfort. If the infection advances, hospitalization and treatment with intravenous antibiotics or even surgery may be needed to clear up pelvic peritonitis and abscesses. In the longterm, PID is a leading cause of infertility, ectopic pregnancy, and chronic pelvic pain. Among women with a history of PID, 20 percent have fertility problems, up to 15 percent experience ectopic pregnancies, and 20 percent suffer from chronic pelvic pain.

STDs and PID can cause scarring and adhesions. Scars and adhesions can push Fallopian tubes out of place, making it difficult or impossible for them to catch an ovum as it bursts from a ripened follicle on the ovary. Or they can occlude, or block, the Fallopian tubes themselves, hampering or preventing an egg from moving down the Fallopian tube and sperm from swimming up to meet it.

Sometimes the blockage is in a place that doesn't allow the fertilized egg to enter the uterus and implant itself properly. The result: an *ectopic pregnancy*. The overwhelming majority of ectopic pregnancies implant in the Fallopian tubes. This can be a life-threatening situation because the growing embryo may burst the tube, leading to massive internal bleeding or even death.

In men STDs can impair sperm production and damage or obstruct the delicate epididymis. As in women, severe cases of STDs can lead to total obstruction of key pathways, like the epididymis, and chronic pain.

How STDs and PID wreak havoc

The most common STDs—and those most responsible for PID and its aftermath, infertility or ectopic pregnancy—are *chlamydial infection* and *gonorrhea*. These infections are caused by the bacteria *Chlamydia trachomatis* and *Neisseria gonorrhoeae*, respectively. When recognized and treated promptly, these infections are easily cured with appropriate antibiotics. If unchecked, these organisms travel easily from the vagina and cervix up the reproductive tract. However, the organisms are not found in nearly one-third of women with PID, although they might have been present in early stages of the infection.

Douching is thought by some to increase the risk of PID by changing the delicate vaginal environment and enhancing the migration of organisms in the lower genital tract into the upper reproductive tract. Pelvic surgeries, such as an abortion or *D&C* (*dilation and curettage*), have been implicated as risk factors for PID. Certainly, these procedures can be a source of adhesions in some patients and contribute to infertility. Age, too, may be a factor: women in their early twenties have a higher incidence of PID than older women. So do those with a history of STDs or multiple sexual partners.

Silent chlamydial infection
Often STDs, in particular, chlamydial infection, don't cause symptoms. Because of this, they can be passed unknowingly countless times between a man and a woman, causing extensive damage. It's often not until you're trying to conceive or you suffer an ectopic pregnancy that their damage is discovered. Because symptoms can be mild or nonexistent, if you have vague abdominal pain or heavy, irregular periods, tell your doctor.

Be sure your doctor tests both you and your partner for *chlamydial infection* at your initial evaluation and later if you're undergoing *in vitro fertilization* (*IVF*) or one of the other assisted reproductive technologies.

One more point: chlamydial infection can have serious consequences in newborns. Babies born to women with active chlamydial infection are subject to infection during passage through the birth canal. They can pick up the organism, which can cause serious eye infection and pneumonia.

Antisperm antibodies

Sometimes the immune system plays a role in infertility. Men and women can actually have an allergic reaction to sperm. Their bodies respond to sperm as foreign substances and produce antibodies to them, in essence, attacking them. (In fact, a man will produce antisperm antibodies when his sperm comes into contact with his blood, such as during an infection. Sperm are normally protected against exposure to a man's own blood.) Among other ways that antisperm antibodies may result in infertility is their ability to cause sperm to clump together, making conception impossible.

The role, if any, of antisperm antibodies in infertility is uncertain and their diagnosis and treatment is controversial. Steroids are used in some cases, but high-dose steroids can be associated with significant risks and there is question about the benefits. Another antisperm antibody controversy is whether they interfere with the implantation and survival of an early embryo. Implantation failure, as it is called, is an area of current active investigation.

Diabetes

Diabetes is a common condition that can affect fertility in both men and women by damaging delicate blood vessels (*microvascular complications*) and nerves (*diabetic neuropathy*).

In men, diabetes can cause *impotence* (*erectile dysfunction*) or *retrograde ejaculation*, the backward movement of semen into the bladder instead of forward out the urethra.

Impotence

As we learned in Chapter 1, achieving and maintaining an erection depends on a healthy supply of blood vessels to the penis and healthy nerves to

Unofficially... Men used to be advised to use a condom during sexual intercourse for several months if their partners had antibodies to their sperm. That's just an old-wives'—or rather, old-doctors'—tale.

signal those blood vessels to open and allow blood to flow into it. Diabetes can impair erectile function in two ways. One is by narrowing the blood vessels to the penis, preventing a flow of enough blood sufficient to engorge the penis and allow it to become or remain erect. Another way is by damaging nerves that signal blood vessels to move blood into the penis. While nearly half of all men with diabetes will experience impotence during their lifetime, medications and treatments are available to help rectify this problem. And, of course, good blood sugar control will help prevent it.

Retrograde ejaculation

During ejaculation, the bladder sphincter closes so that semen can be expelled out the urethra. Diabetic neuropathy can damage the bladder sphincter nerves, causing it not to close properly. The result: Semen takes the path of least resistance backwards into the bladder. The result is little or no sperm in the ejaculate.

Diabetes and women

Uncontrolled diabetes can affect a woman's ability to conceive and maintain a pregnancy. Sometimes diabetes will prevent ovulation or implantation, or cause such an early miscarriage that a pregnancy goes unnoticed.

If you or your partner has diabetes and you are thinking about trying to conceive, be certain to get your blood glucose under control. If you're having trouble conceiving, complications of diabetes may be the problem, so be certain your doctor checks for evidence of diabetic causes.

Smoking

It's fairly well known that cigarette smoking increases the risk of spontaneous abortion and low birth-weight babies. But did you know that smoking can increase the time to conception, as well? Researchers aren't sure why, but they think that cigarette smoking reduces some types of estrogen production and may deplete egg supply. Smoking can also hasten menopause, which can shorten the amount of time you have to conceive.

It's already known that smoking interferes with Fallopian tube motility, embryo cleavage, blastocyst formation, and implantation. (See Chapter 1 for more information about early embryo development.) Tobacco smoke chemicals, which could be toxic to sperm, have also been found in cervical mucus.

Women who smoke are also less likely to have success with in vitro fertilization than nonsmokers. And just because you don't smoke doesn't mean you haven't been affected by it. Women whose mothers smoked during pregnancy are less likely to produce a live birth. And men who smoke produce fewer and less healthy sperm. On average, smokers have sperm counts that are 15 percent lower than those of nonsmokers.

Bright Idea
Here's yet another reason for quitting smoking: a small study found that sperm counts rose dramatically—50 percent to 800 percent—in men who stopped smoking.

Alcohol and mind-altering drugs

Alcohol and mind-altering drugs (marijuana; cocaine; stimulants such as amphetamines, phencyclidine, and "angel dust"; and depressants, such as barbiturates, tranquilizers, and heroin) can adversely affect the reproductive function of both men and women.

In women, marijuana, for example, can shorten the menstrual cycle, in particular the luteal phase. In men, alcohol and illicit drugs can lower sperm counts and impair sperm quality, upset hormonal balance, and cause impotence. While it's uncertain how much of these substances must be used before seeing harmful effects, men with borderline fertility problems would be wise not to risk further impairment.

Diethylstilbestrol (DES)

Diethylstilbestrol (DES) has been found to impair fertility in the sons and daughters of women who had been given this synthetic estrogen in the 1950s to prevent miscarriage. Studies have shown that some DES daughters have a wide range of cervical, uterine, and tubal abnormalities. Any one of these can prevent conception or lead to ectopic pregnancy, miscarriage, and premature labor.

In men, prenatal DES exposure is thought to cause diminished sperm production, epididymal cysts, obstructions of the epididymis and vas deferens, and undescended testes (*cryptorchidism*), a condition in which the testes have not descended normally into the scrotum during fetal development.

Athletic activity and weight

Young female athletes—especially those who are very underweight and have little body fat—are at risk for reproductive dysfunction. In fact, the percent of body fat may influence both the onset and maintenance of ovulation.

While some aspects of physical activity, weight, and age, and their interrelationships with reproduction are debated, one fact is clear: extreme or rapid weight loss can disrupt ovulation in women who have had regular cycles. For example, young women with *anorexia nervosa* have impaired hypothalamus function. Their serum contains almost undetectable amounts of the hormones FSH and LH, which regulate ovulation.

Watch Out!
Frequent use of hot tubs and working near pizza ovens have been found to cause infertility in men.

Just as being too thin is harmful, being overweight or obese is, too. It can affect hormonal signals in both men and women. In women, extra weight can increase insulin levels, which may cause the ovaries to overproduce male hormones and stop releasing eggs. Being overweight also contributes to the development of diabetes, a risk factor for infertility. Fat can also produce hormone changes, which can affect ovulation in women and sperm production in men.

Female factor infertility

As we saw in Chapter 1, the female reproductive system is quite complex. Its many different organs and intricate and delicate set of hormones are subject to a variety of problems.

Many factors can affect a woman's ability to ovulate, conceive, or carry a pregnancy to term. Often, more than one factor is to blame. In fact, in 25 percent of infertile couples, more than one factor contributes to the impaired fertility.

For convenience, sometimes doctors group female infertility problems into categories, such as structural, hormonal, or immunological disorders. More often, they divide the causes into four categories by location:

- Cervical
- Tubal
- Ovarian
- Uterine

Unfortunately, sometimes more than one category is involved. Just because a problem in one of these categories is identified, it doesn't mean you should stop looking for others. Be sure your doctor rules out other likely causes, including male factor infertility.

Cervical factors

As we saw in Chapter 1, the cervix is a vital component in the female reproductive system. It is the conduit through which sperm must first pass from the vagina into the uterus, up the Fallopian tube, and, it is hoped, to an awaiting egg. Good-quality cervical mucus is essential, too, for sperm to survive and pass through this first hurdle on the journey to conception. Here are some cervical abnormalities that can impair conception or lead to miscarriage:

- Malformations of the cervical canal, such as those seen in DES daughters.

- Malpositioning of the cervix, which is very rare.

- Infections, which can produce poor quality, thick cervical mucus that can restrict or prevent sperm movement.

- Injury from medical procedures, such as cryosurgery, cone biopsy, conization, or cauterization, which are often performed after abnormal Pap smear results.

Tubal factors

Timesaver
Because endometriosis tends to run in families, tell your doctor if your mother or sisters had symptoms or were diagnosed with the disease.

Damaged or malfunctioning Fallopian tubes account for 20 to 35 percent of the infertility cases treated. These abnormalities will prevent eggs from ever reaching the approaching sperm. The tubes may be blocked or immobilized by scar tissue, which makes it impossible for them to move and to pick up eggs.

Tubal obstruction and/or blockages and immobilization are often caused by scars and adhesions from previous infections, inflammation, and surgery. (See above for more about STDs and PID and their role in causing tubal disorders.)

Any number of conditions or procedures could also narrow or totally block the Fallopian tubes, hamper their natural movement or that of their fimbriae, or impair their ability to secrete essential fluids. For example, women who have had pelvic surgery for a ruptured appendix, ectopic pregnancy, fibroid removal, or an ovarian cyst, are at risk for tubal disease. Likewise, women who have used an IUD or had two or more induced abortions may also be at increased risk for tubal disease.

Here are other possible causes of tubal disease:

- Infection—whether apparent to you or not.

- Miscarriage

- Endometriosis

- Tubal sterilization

Ovarian factors

Ovarian disorders can prevent the development and ovulation of viable ova. Irregular or abnormal ovulation accounts for approximately 25 percent— some estimates place it as high as 33 percent—of all female infertility cases. Tell your doctor if you have abnormal periods, such as heavy flow or cramps, or irregularly occurring periods. These may signal ovarian dysfunction.

As we learned in Chapter 1, the primary ovarian function, ovulation, is tightly regulated by hormones. Any impairment in hypothalamic, pituitary, or ovarian function can lead to *anovulation,* which is the absence of egg release, or to infrequent ovulation.

Other endocrine, or hormone-producing, system disorders that do not control ovulation directly can also cause infertility. For example, thyroid disease, hypercortisolism, and diabetes are frequently linked to ovulatory dysfunction. And, of course, how old you are has a strong impact on ovarian function. The younger you are the greater your chance to conceive. The older, the lower your chances.

Some less common medical causes of ovarian factor infertility are congenital abnormalities; polycystic ovarian disease, which is common in women who do not ovulate; endometriosis; and some drugs.

Uterine factors

Uterine factors can interfere with fertility by:

- Causing structural problems, such as fibroids, polyps, or adhesions, which provide a poor environment.

- Preventing implantation of a fertilized egg into the uterine wall.

- Preventing embryo implantation.

Here are some conditions and problems that can cause uterine factor infertility.

Endometriosis, a condition in which normally shed uterine tissue migrates outside the uterus is another major cause of infertility. Endometrial tissue is sometimes found on the ovaries, Fallopian tubes, and on the bladder and bowel. As many as 35 percent of women who undergo laparoscopy during infertility work-up are found to have endometriosis. Doctors have known for some time that endometriosis tends to run in families. But, recently, investigators have actually found a specific chromosomal abnormalities in women with endometriosis.

Although endometriosis can be symptomless, the most common signs of endometriosis are:

- painful menstrual cramps.

- diarrhea or painful bowel movements, especially around the time of your period.

Unofficially...
A sperm is one-thousandth of an inch long. It must swim six inches to reach a mature egg. That's equivalent to a man swimming 100 miles!

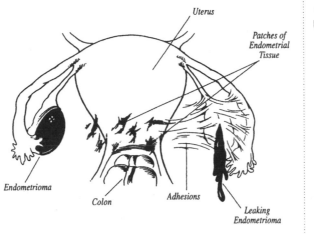

Uterus

Patches of
Endometrial
Tissue

Endometrioma

Colon

Adhesions

Leaking
Endometrioma

← **Note!**
Endometriosis.

- painful sexual intercourse.

- congenital deformities, such as a so-called double (*bicornuate*) uterus and a divided (*septate*) uterus.

Tumors, especially polyps and fibroids, which are noncancerous growths, can distort or reduce the uterus's size and capacity and interfere with the endometrium's blood supply and nutrition. Fibroids are quite common. It is their location and size that determines whether or not they'll interfere with your conceiving, embryo implantation, or carrying to term. There are three types of fibroids:

- Submucosal, which grow inside the uterine cavity, can erode the endometrium making it unable to prepare itself for embryo implantation.

- Intramural, which grow inside the uterus's muscle wall, may not hamper your conceiving, but if they grow big enough to disturb blood supply, they can interfere fetal growth.

■ Subserosal, which grow on or protrude into the outer surface of the uterus, can compress the Fallopian tubes, interfering with their ability to pick up an ovulated egg.

Other endometrial disorders, such infection, or scarring from incomplete abortions or procedures such as curettage following childbirth, may also adversely affect your chances of conceiving.

Male factor infertility

Infertility is not for women only. About 30 percent of infertility cases involve a male factor and about 20 percent involve factors from both partners. With these statistics, the male partner is either the sole or a contributing cause of infertility in half of the infertile couples. Like those of female infertility, male causes of infertility are categorized, usually into seminal and structural abnormalities.

Seminal abnormalities

Seminal abnormalities include low or poor sperm production. Both the quantity and the quality of sperm are important for conception to occur.

When no sperm are found in the ejaculate, the condition is called *azoospermia*; a low sperm count is called *oligospermia*. If too few sperm are ejaculated during sexual intercourse, the chances of a viable sperm meeting an egg are greatly reduced.

Not only is the number of sperm important, but so is the quality. Sperm quality is judged according to their motility (ability to move) and their morphology (structure). Without good motility, sperm cannot make that long swim up to an awaiting egg. If damaged, they can't swim properly or penetrate an egg.

Unofficially...
New research is finding the cause in more and more cases of unexplained infertility. For example, upwards of 18 percent of men with unexplained oligospermia have been found to have an abnormality on their Y chromosomes.

Deformed sperm come in many shapes and sizes. Those with more than one head or tail, or too long or too short a head or tail, cannot fertilize an egg.

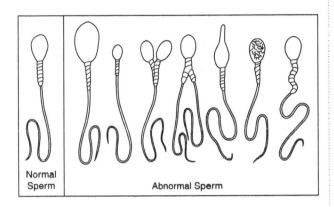

Normal
Sperm

Abnormal Sperm

← **Note!**
Normal and abnormal sperm morphology. Abnormal sperm shape is one male factor cause of infertility.

Structural abnormalities

Male infertility can be caused by structural (sometimes called anatomical) anomalies that are present at birth, are complications of illness or surgery, or develop over time. The main male factors for infertility include the following:

■ *Varicocele*, which is a network of dilated varicose veins in the scrotum, is the most common cause of infertility in men. More than 90 percent of varicoceles are found on the left side.

■ Undescended testes (*cryptorchidism*) is a congenital deformity in which the testes do not descend normally from the abdomen into the scrotum during fetal development. If the testes remain in the abdomen too long, sperm production is impaired.

- Surgical complications, sometimes after hernia repair, prostate or bladder neck operations, and testicular cancer surgery.

- Obstruction of the vas deferens or epididymis, which impairs the sperm's ability to travel normally into the penis during ejaculation. A man can be born with these obstructions or get them after an infection or surgery. Sometimes, however, their cause is unknown.

- Voluntary sterilization (*vasectomy*), in which the vas deferens is closed off, preventing sperm from mixing with the ejaculate.

Medical disorders

Several medical conditions can also harm male fertility. The most common are infections and injury. In addition, cystic fibrosis, sickle-cell disease, and renal disease can impair a man's ability to father a child.

And, as we talked about earlier, a variety of drugs and environmental agents can hamper male fertility.

Infections

Several medical conditions, in particular, infections, can affect a man's ability to produce a child. These include: *prostatitis* (an infection of the prostate gland), genital infection (including STDs), and mumps after puberty. In general, these infections can lead to scarring and obstruction of the epididymis, sperm ducts, or testes.

Another common infection that can seriously impair fertility is *epididymitis,* an infection in the epididymis. Although highly treatable with antibiotics, when left unattended, epididymitis can cause obstruction that prevents sperm from leaving the testes.

Watch Out!
Just because your partner may have gotten another woman pregnant does not mean that he is still fertile. Sperm quantity and quality can change dramatically over time. Make sure he has a current semen analysis.

In fact, any infection or fever can impair sperm development and affect the ability to conceive for three months! So if your doctor orders sperm analysis, don't forget that one test result is not always conclusive.

Testicular trauma or torsion

Testicular trauma or torsion can injure the testes and impair their function. Torsion is a condition in which a testis twists on the cord that attaches it to the body. The sudden interruption of blood flow to and from the testicle causes dramatic and painful swelling. Surgical correction is usually very successful at saving the testis. But, if untreated, the testis will shrivel and die.

Medications, toxins, and illicit drugs

A variety of drugs—therapeutic and illicit—can have detrimental, and sometimes devastating, effects on male fertility. These can range from impotence to sterility. In addition, exposure to environmental and occupational toxins can impair testicular function. These include the following:

- Chemotherapeutic agents
- Radiotherapy
- Anabolic steroids
- Common prescription medications, in particular those given to control high blood pressure (spironolactone, beta-blockers), ulcers (cimetidine), ulcerative colitis (sulfasalazine), depression (MAO inhibitors), seizures (dilantin), and infections (nitrofurantoin)
- Toxins, including Agent Orange, anesthetic gases, benzene, lead, cadmium, mercury, manganese, and dibromochloropropane (DBCP) used in pesticides

Myths and misconceptions about infertility

It's important to remember that in about 85 to 90 percent of infertility cases a specific cause or causes can be found and treated. Despite the best evaluations, no cause for infertility is found in the remaining 10 to 15 percent or so of infertile couples. Unexplained infertility has been responsible for some of the most common and persistent myths and misconceptions about infertility.

Myth #1: Stress is a common cause of infertility.

Every infertile couple has heard the "relax and you'll get pregnant" line, or "just take a vacation." Not only is this incorrect, but it implies that it's the woman's fault because she is too stressed or uptight to become pregnant. We do know definitely that infertility does causes stress, but there is scant evidence that stress is a major cause of infertility.

In fact, most of the so-called evidence about stress and infertility is anecdotal. We all know of cases where women try to conceive for years and years, take huge doses of fertility drugs, undergo countless surgical procedures, and nothing happens. Then they stop all treatment, and lo and behold, they become pregnant—presumably because they stopped trying so hard and "relaxed." But, statistically speaking this outcome is the exception, not the rule.

That's not to say that stress doesn't affect fertility in certain ways. The ability of a man to achieve and maintain an erection, as well as the frequency of intercourse can all be adversely affected by stress. Also, stress can throw off a woman's menstrual cycle. But that is usually temporary, and fertility drugs work very nicely to regulate a woman's cycle.

Unofficially...
Until the nineteenth century, infertility was always blamed on the woman. Finally, in 1864, Dr. Curling, a British physician, wrote in a medical textbook that infertility could be caused by the man.

Just the facts

- Under age thirty a woman has a 20 percent chance of conceiving each month. By age forty, her chances of conceiving drop to only 5 percent each month.

- Pelvic inflammatory disease—often silent, often devastating—is a leading cause of infertility, ectopic pregnancy, and chronic pelvic pain.

- Smoking can deplete egg stores in woman and delay time to conception. It can reduce sperm production in men.

- Studies have shown that some DES daughters may have a wide range of cervical, uterine, and tubal abnormalities.

- Being too thin or too fat can impair a woman's ability to conceive and maintain a pregnancy to term.

Finding the Problem

PART II

GET THE SCOOP ON...
When to consult a doctor ▪ Finding a good
fertility specialist ▪ Taking control of your
treatment ▪ When to switch doctors

Dealing with Doctors

To overcome a fertility problem, you and your partner will need to undergo testing, and most likely one or both of you will undergo some form of treatment—be it hormonal, surgical, or both. But first, you need know what the problem is—or at least be able to rule out certain conditions. The best way to do this is to consult a fertility specialist.

Finding the right doctor for you

Many women naturally gravitate to their regular OB/GYNs when they think they have a fertility problem. This may seem like the logical choice to you. After all, your OB/GYN knows you and has probably been handling your contraceptive needs and gynecological problems for many years. While this may be okay as a preliminary step, seeing your regular OB/GYN is ultimately not the best choice unless he or she is a qualified fertility specialist. Most OB/GYNs, do not have the advanced training in infertility necessary to effectively diagnose and treat many of the more serious infertility problems.

Chapter 3

Infertility is a couple's problem that requires specialized knowledge of both the male and female reproductive systems. This is especially true since at least half the time, male factor infertility is a primary or secondary cause of a couple's inability to conceive. Some doctors say they are fertility specialists regardless of their postgraduate or specialized training. Remember, just because doctors advertise themselves as fertility specialists doesn't mean they are.

Bright Idea
If you're already seeing a fertility specialist and your partner is not, ask for a referral for your partner. You'll be certain that way you'll both be on the same track and your doctors can consult with each other about your case.

What is a fertility specialist?

A fertility specialist should be a licensed medical doctor who has extensive postgraduate training in reproductive medicine, and usually reproductive endocrinology and reproductive surgery, as well. Usually OB/GYNs and urologists are the ones who ultimately become fertility specialists. Depending on your particular problem and needed treatment, you and your partner may see one or more of these fertility specialists.

Obstetrician-Gynecologists (OB/GYNs)

Physicians who are board certified in the surgical specialties of obstetrics (the management of pregnancy and childbirth) and gynecology (the diagnosis and treatment of the female reproductive system). They may or may not have extensive training in infertility. Many OB/GYNs devote a large portion of their time to obstetrics.

Gynecologists

Doctors who have usually been trained as OB/GYNs but have chosen to specialize in gynecology.

Reproductive Endocrinologists (REs)

These are OB/GYNs who have completed a fellowship in reproductive endocrinology. This involves three years of intensive training in infertility, focussing on the role of hormones in reproduction. To become board certified, they must then pass special examinations conducted by the American Board of Obstetrics and Gynecology.

Reproductive Surgeons

REs who have additional advanced training in microsurgery, and are usually trained in the assisted reproductive technologies such as in vitro fertilization (IVF). They are sometimes referred to as reproductive surgeons. Reproductive surgeons can be urologists as well as OB/GYNs.

Urologists

Physicians who specialize in the diagnosis and treatment of the urinary tract in men and women, as well as the male reproductive organs. Urologists are also qualified surgeons. They may or may not have had advanced training in the diagnosis and treatment of male infertility.

Andrologists

Physicians, usually urologists, who specialize in the male reproductive system and male hormones. Many andrologists also specialize in infertility.

What to look for in a doctor

Finding a good doctor is not always easy. Nor should you expect it to be. Your success in overcoming infertility depends heavily upon the doctor you choose. So you should be prepared to devote some time and care in choosing your specialist. Some people balk at the idea of questioning prospective physicians—they may feel intimidated or they just may not want to go through the effort. If that describes you or your partner, ask yourselves this question. Would you buy a new house without researching and carefully inspecting it? Or a car, for

Watch Out!
Be wary of
doctors who
guarantee that
they will help
you get preg-
nant. No doctor
can or should
guarantee this.

that matter? Your medical care should be even more important. You'll be investing a lot of money and time in your doctor. Your chances of fulfilling your hopes and dreams for a family depend, to a large extent, on this doctor. That's why it's important to choose this person very carefully.

There are basically three important things you need to look for in a fertility specialist: credentials, convenience, and compatibility.

Credentials

You should always ask about the doctor's post-graduate training. Some doctors say they're fertility specialists but lack the necessary training.

Fertility specialists should be either *board certified* or *board eligible.* A physician who is a board certified reproductive endocrinologist first has to have completed a residency in obstetrics and gynecology. She or he then has to take a three-year fellowship in reproductive endocrinology, and pass both written and oral exams. Those who have done all the above except taking or passing their oral exams are considered board eligible reproductive endocrinologists. Once they pass their oral exams, they become board certified.

While there are about 28,000 OB/GYNs in the United States, only about 500 are board certified, and another 800 board eligible, in reproductive endocrinology. Most of these subspecialists practice in large cities or medical centers.

There are several ways of checking a doctor's credentials:

- Contact RESOLVE, a not-for-profit national support, education, and advocacy organization for infertile men and women. Local chapters of RESOLVE keep an up-to-date list of fertility specialists that includes information about their qualifications.

- Call your county medical society. Local county medical societies have directories of physicians that give information such as medical school attended, year of graduation, and board certification or eligibility in a specialty or subspecialty. You can usually find these directories in your local public library.

- Ask the doctor. You can ask the doctor directly about his or her qualifications, or check the diplomas on the wall. You can always double-check by calling the medical school or hospital where the doctor says he or she was trained.

- Check with the appropriate medical board, such as the American Board of Obstetrics and Gynecology or the American Board of Urology.

Convenience

Infertility treatment is a major inconvenience in most peoples' lives. Therefore, it is helpful to find a doctor who is conveniently located, has convenient hours and offers other amenities. Here's a list of convenience factors you might want to consider:

- *Location.* Not everyone has enough qualified doctors to choose from to be picky about location. But if you live in an area with many fertility specialists, location is something to consider, especially if you are working. Infertility testing and treatment can be very time consuming. For example, you may have to go in for blood tests, sonograms, or inseminations several days in a row. Getting away from work in the middle of the day for doctors' appointments can be tricky business. So the location of your doctor's

Bright Idea
Ask what percentage of the doctor's practice is devoted to infertility, and what percentage is obstetrics and gynecology. Fertility specialists should devote most, if not all, of their time to infertility patients. And look around the waiting room. If you see mostly pregnant patients, chances are the doctor is primarily practicing obstetrics and may not have the necessary time to devote to infertility.

practice can be very important. On the other hand, you don't want to sacrifice quality of care for a convenient location.

- *Office hours.* Flexible office hours can be extremely useful. If you aren't always able to get away from work for doctors' appointments, a doctor with early morning hours or evening hours might be best for you. Weekend coverage and weekend hours can sometimes be important. Be sure to discuss scheduling issues with the doctor ahead of time.

- *Phone hours.* Ask about phone hours. Some doctors have special hours set aside for patients to call about test results or other important medical matters. You should feel free to call your doctor whether or not there are special phone hours, but be brief, both out of consideration for your doctor and the other patients who may need to reach him or her. Many doctors don't charge for short calls. However, if your phone calls become too time-consuming, your doctor will most likely charge you an amount pre-determined by your insurance policy. Sometimes phone calls are handled by your doctor's nurse or other assistants. This can be fine, especially if they're familiar with your case.

- *Type of practice—group or solo.* Seeing a doctor in a group practice solves some problems, such as weekend coverage. These groups also tend to have more flexible hours than solo practices, as well. However, while you're always guaranteed to have a physician available at all times, you probably won't always get to see the doctor of your choice. A solo practice provides consistency of approach, continuity of care, and regular contact with the same physician. But he sometimes cannot addresss the issue of weekend hours.

■ *Help with insurance.* Since infertility treatment can be incredibly expensive, a physician's willingness to help you with medical insurance issues can be crucial. In fact, some fertility specialists hire people just to help their patients— and themselves—with insurance matters. Your doctor should be willing to provide the insurer with the necessary information about your case, and his or her staff should be willing to help you fill out the appropriate forms. But keep in mind that your health insurance policy is a contract between you and your insurer. Whether or not you get reimbursed is ultimately up to your insurance company, not your doctor.

■ *On-site lab and other equipment.* Ideally, your doctor will have the necessary equipment in or near his or her office so that you don't have to run all around town for various tests. Most reproductive endocrinologists will have the necessary equipment to do routine and sometimes advanced tests and procedures. Some doctors may not have room for all the necessary equipment, but they should be able to refer you to convenient nearby facilities.

Compatibility

Compatibility with one's doctor, while very important, can be very difficult to assess. And you certainly can't assess it until you actually go and see the doctor. You may instantly bond with your doctor and then, after a few months, feel differently. Or you may not take to him or her right away, but as

Moneysaver
Get all the information you can about a doctor *before* your first appointment. After checking his or her credentials, call the office manager or nurse and ask about office hours, coverage, fees, and insurance plans. If you don't like what you hear, don't make or keep any appointment with that doctor.

you become more comfortable with each other, you may develop a compatible doctor-patient relationship.

Compatibility is not the same thing as liking or loving. You just have to have a good working relationship, one in which you and your viewpoints are respected, and one in which you participate equally in the major decisions about your treatment.

What about charisma?

Some people think that personality counts when it comes to choosing a doctor, but does it really? A very competent doctor may not be someone you'd want to sit next to on a twelve-hour plane flight, while a charming doctor may be totally incompetent. So while personality counts to some extent, it shouldn't be overestimated as a major criterion for choosing a doctor.

Looking for Dr. Right

Now that you know what to look for in a doctor, how do you go about finding the right doctor for you? Keep in mind that there is no such thing as the best doctor. There are many good, competent doctors, and your job is to find one that is well suited to your needs.

There are many ways to find a good fertility specialist, and you should probably not depend on one source. The first step is to collect names. The second step is to check their credentials to make certain they are, in fact, qualified fertility specialists. If several names come up repeatedly as good (or bad) doctors, that will help you narrow down your list. To collect a preliminary list of names, here's where to go:

- *RESOLVE.* Described earlier, RESOLVE is the largest organization for infertile men and women in the nation, and is probably your best bet for finding a good fertility specialist. In addition, join RESOLVE (or other similar groups) to get the inside scoop on local fertility doctors.

- *Friends.* It's a good idea to ask friends who have experienced infertility for recommendations. Keep in mind that a recommendation by a friend, however, is not always an indication of a doctor's qualification as a fertility specialist or even good nonspecialist. Just because a doctor helped your friend get pregnant doesn't mean he or she is the appropriate doctor for you and your particular problem. Physician friends can be especially helpful since not only might they know the names of some good fertility specialists, they can also check out a doctor's credentials *and* reputation.

- *Your personal physicians.* Your doctors—especially OB/GYNs, internists, and family physicians—can all be excellent sources of referral. They can also give you feedback on the doctors you're already considering.

- *The American Society for Reproductive Medicine (ASRM).* Formerly called the American Fertility Society, ASRM is an organization of professionals interested in reproductive medicine. ASRM can provide you with the names of its members in your location. But since professionals from many fields related to infertility can become ASRM members, you'll need to further check out their credentials and particular fields of expertise and interests.

Bright Idea
Before committing yourself to a particular fertility specialist, make an appointment for a preliminary consultation. It's a good way to assess compatibility before you undergo any extensive testing or treatment.

Moneysaver
Go to as many infertility talks or symposia as you can. You'll have a chance to meet doctors informally and ask them questions for free.

- *Local hospitals.* You can call your local hospital or medical center to find out which doctors on staff specialize in infertility. Again, you should check out their credentials further.

- *Yellow pages.* If you have no other choice, you may want to consult the Yellow Pages. But a name or an ad in the Yellow Pages is no guarantee that the doctor is indeed a competent fertility specialist.

Once you have the names of several good fertility specialists, check to see which physicians are covered by your insurance plan. Then start calling for appointments. It's best to make appointments with several different doctors for consultations, since you won't immediately know if the doctor you've initially chosen to see is the right one for you. If you find one you like, you can cancel the other appointments if you give them enough notice. However, it may be a good idea to keep the appointments for second opinions or as alternatives if the first doctor doesn't work out.

Common obstacles to consulting a fertility doctor

If you're still hesitant about consulting a fertility specialist, it may be helpful to explore some of the reasons why some couples wait month after frustrating month before picking up the phone and calling a specialist, while others make an appointment the minute they suspect a problem.

One of the most common reasons people put off seeking infertility treatment is denial. Most of us have a hard time admitting to ourselves that we can't do what everyone else seems to do with ease—reproduce. It's also easy to be in denial when there are no physical symptoms present. Most people go to doctors because they have physical pain or discomfort, but this is rarely the case with infertility. Although infertility is a physical disorder, most patients do not suffer physically. Rather, their suffering is primarily emotional—caused by feeling deprived of having children. Because there is usually no pressing need for physical symptom relief, people suffering from infertility can postpone going to the doctor indefinitely. But this form of denial can't last forever. When their emotional pain or frustration becomes too great, they seek medical treatment.

When a person consults a fertility doctor, it's an admission that something is probably wrong with his or her reproductive system. That person is then faced with the possibility of not only potentially painful and expensive diagnostic tests and treatment, but the more painful possibility of never being able to have a biological child. But remember, if you delay consulting a doctor, you'll be wasting precious time. And you won't be any closer to conceiving.

Many people also find the label "infertility" very stigmatizing and embarrassing. Both men and women often see infertility as a reflection of their sexuality—a man may feel less of a man, and a woman less of a woman. Men tend to see their inability to impregnate their wives as a direct reflection on their masculinity—they equate fertility with virility, and infertility with impotence. While the ability to have and maintain an erection is an advantage when it comes to getting a woman pregnant, it's not a necessity. Many infertile couples conceive through artificial insemination with the husband's sperm, regardless of whether the husband is impotent. (See the discussion on artificial insemination in Chapter 5.)

Timesaver
Call at least one week ahead of time to make sure your new doctor has received any past medical records. If they haven't, make sure they get there before you do—even if you have to get them yourself.

Some men are so embarrassed by infertility—even when it's their partner who has the underlying physical problem—that they're reluctant to consult a specialist. Some are afraid that if they consult a fertility doctor, they will have to discuss their sex lives with a total stranger, often another man, and they find that prospect threatening.

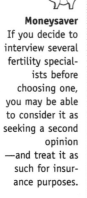

Moneysaver
If you decide to interview several fertility specialists before choosing one, you may be able to consider it as seeking a second opinion —and treat it as such for insurance purposes.

Making the most of your consultation

When you finally do get to the point of seeing a specialist, you want the consultation to be as useful and informative as possible. The following suggestions will help you get the most out of both an initial consultation and subsequent office visits.

- Bring your partner. It's important both medically and emotionally to involve your significant other right from the beginning.
- Write down your questions ahead of time and bring them with you whenever you see the doctor.
- Both you and your partner should take notes and jot down any questions or concerns that occur to you during the consultation.

Not being taken seriously

There is another obstacle to initiating infertility treatment many couples face, and that is going first to a doctor who does not think they have a real problem. When a couple finally consults a doctor about infertility, they expect something to be done about it. The woman is usually ready to begin her infertility workup so that her problem can quickly be diagnosed and treated. But some OB/GYNs may not take the couple seriously. This is another reason it's important to see a fertility specialist.

A related problem that many older women face is that despite the evidence that infertility increases after the age of thirty, many doctors treat their older patients in much the same way they treat their younger ones. They follow the general rule that you wait one full year before initiating an infertility workup or treatment. Most fertility specialists, however, believe that a woman over the age of thirty who has not conceived in six months probably should start an infertility work-up, and any woman over thirty-five should definitely consult a specialist after six months. If your convinced you have a fertility problem and your doctor isn't, find another doctor—someone at least willing to explore the possibility that you have something wrong.

Taking charge of your infertility treatment

Once you've settled on a good fertility specialist, you may be tempted to sit back and let the doctor do all the work. But infertility, like any important issue in your life, requires you to make important decisions. While many people prefer to have their doctor call all the shots (since the doctor is, after all, the expert), keep in mind that you're ultimately responsible for your own health care. This, however, does not mean that you become your own doctor. It *does* mean that you become an active participant in your treatment. You and your physician form a partnership, based on mutual cooperation and respect. As an equal partner in that relationship, you have important responsibilities. For example, it's up to you to provide accurate information to your doctor and ask questions when you don't understand something.

> **66**
>
> As an informed patient, I think I was able to add to my treatment. I think that we had quicker success because I was participating. I had some good ideas about my own treatment and my doctor was never threatened by it. He was always receptive to my suggestions.
> —Karen, a thirty-eight-year-old administrator.
>
> **99**

Infertility treatment requires your full participation. You have to constantly evaluate and re-evaluate the situation so you can make the best decisions for yourself. This can only be done with the help and support of your doctor and, ideally, your partner.

Becoming medically knowledgeable about infertility is perhaps the best way to work positively with your doctor toward your ultimate goal—achieving a successful pregnancy. Remember, knowledge is power. And most doctors will appreciate an involved, well-informed patient. Here are some ways that can help:

Moneysaver
Many doctors charge by the page to copy medical records. Request that the records go to you, and you can make as many copies as you want more cheaply on your own. Not only will you save money, you'll have a full set of records for your own use.

- Keep a copy of all your medical records at home.

- If you have any questions or concerns about tests or treatments, call your doctor. Make sure all your questions get answered.

- Always weigh the pros and cons, the risks and benefits of every test, drug, and treatment your doctor recommends.

- Read everything you can on infertility. Go to bookstores, medical libraries, public libraries, and the Internet.

- Become an expert on your and/or your partner's particular problem.

- Go to RESOLVE meetings and infertility seminars and symposia.

- Join a RESOLVE or other support group.

- Talk to as many people as you can who have had or currently have fertility problems.

- Trust your instincts. If you have doubts about your doctor, find another one.

The doctor-patient relationship

Your relationship with your fertility doctor is a partnership based on mutual cooperation and it should be a smooth one. After all, you both are working toward the same goal. But, as in every relationship, there are times when things don't go so smoothly. If you have a difference of opinion with your doctor, discuss it with him and try to resolve the issue.

You might feel intimidated about discussing your differences. But keep in mind that you have nothing to lose and a lot to gain. Discussing these issues can help your doctor better understand you and your needs. But if you find that you and your doctor repeatedly have unresolved differences, you may want to consider finding a new doctor.

Switching doctors or doctor hopping

Infertility patients are notorious for doctor shopping and doctor hopping. Patients often switch doctors if they feel their doctors can no longer help them. When conflicts cannot be resolved, or you believe your doctor can't help you conceive, it may be time to change doctors.

How can you tell if your doctor won't be able to help you conceive? If you feel that you aren't making progress—that you're no closer to a pregnancy or a clear understanding of why you're not getting pregnant after a reasonable period of time—it's time to move on to another doctor, or at least get a second opinion. Whether or not you stay with your doctor or even continue treatment varies from patient to patient. It depends on your age, diagnosis, prognosis, and emotional and financial limits. What is shouldn't depend on is false hope, or unrealistic expectations about your doctor's abilities. No fertility specialist—no matter how famous

❝

We had lots of discussions where we disagreed with our doctor, asked questions, or wanted to try something different. She's really met all our questions or disagreements with solid evidence for what she's doing. She wanted to do a laparoscopy and I said I didn't want to do that right away. She said that was fine—we'd do it when I felt ready for it.
—Julie, a thirty-five-year-old teacher

❞

or well-qualified—can help every patient. Sometimes even the best doctor can miss some subtle aspect of a medical condition. That is why second opinions can, at times, be extremely helpful to both you and your doctor.

Countless patients have wasted considerable time and money by sticking with their OB/GYNs—or even fertility specialists—when they should have moved on to another doctor. On the other hand, skipping from doctor to doctor can be counterproductive. It may take a doctor many months or even years to help you achieve a pregnancy. What is important is that you feel that you are making progress, that another piece of the puzzle has been found, and that different treatment methods are tried.

Bright Idea
Make an appointment periodically just to talk to your doctor so you can both reevaluate your situation and discuss your options.

Just the facts

- If you're seeing your regular OB/GYN, it's time to move on to a qualified reproductive endocrinologist.

- Shop around until you find a doctor who has the right credentials, has a convenient location and hours, and with whom you feel compatible.

- Take charge of your fertility treatment—read, ask questions, and communicate with your doctor about your concerns and suggestions.

- Get a second opinion if either you or your doctor feel it is warranted.

- Switch doctors if you feel your doctor has not given you the care you deserve or if you feel you're making no progress with your doctor.

Chapter 4

GET THE SCOOP ON...
Testing—what's necessary and what's not ▪
Simple self-tests ▪ Why the man must be tested
from the start ▪ Making diagnostic tests as
painless as possible

The Basic Infertility Workup

You've read it a dozen times already in this *Unofficial Guide*, but we'll say it again: Infertility is a *couple's* problem. It's not only because in nearly half of couples experiencing infertility an impairment is found in both partners, but because the road to fertility must be a joint project.

The first step is to find out what's wrong—a process that must involve both of you looking for causes right from the start. And it's a step more easily taken when both of you are in sync philosophically and emotionally.

Often conception depends less on how fertile one partner is than on how compatible—reproductively speaking—the couple is. Your fertility may not be completely up to par, but you might not have much trouble conceiving if your partner's highly fertile. But if both of you have even a moderate fertility problem, however, the chances of conceiving are considerably less. And if one of you has a significant problem and the other a moderate problem, just correcting the moderate problem may not be enough.

Getting ready

Before embarking on a quest for the reason(s) why you're not conceiving, you and your partner should consider separately and then discuss together what lies ahead. Ask yourselves: "What do I(we) want?" "What am I(we) prepared to do?" Of course, circumstances—whether physical, emotional, or even financial—change. So what you decide today doesn't have to be written in stone. You can, and probably will, change your mind. But having some idea of what you're willing to undergo will help you set up a plan of action and a timetable. This puts you in control and will help relieve anxiety.

As we said in the previous chapter, ask questions: "What is this test designed to show?" "What is the next step or steps after this test result is in?" "Will there be more tests?" "What treatment options do we have?" Of course, always ask: "Is this test necessary?" "Will it hurt?" "How long will it take?" There's nothing more irritating than to go in for a test only to find out that it'll take longer than you anticipated, so you'll miss work. Or that the test makes you so uncomfortable you couldn't possibly do anything else that day—or the next.

Remember, *you* decide what tests you take and, ultimately, what treatments you accept. At the same time, these decisions may impact on how rapidly and accurately a diagnosis is made and how successful treatment is.

Reasonable expectations

Keep in mind that infertility is unlike other physical conditions. Uncovering its cause involves two patients, not just one. And, unlike other disorders, diagnosing its cause can easily take several months... more than a year. Infertility also differs from other diseases in that some tests require following a schedule and coordination—one and/or both of you must do something on a specific day. Many of these "must dos" involve the intimate aspects of your life—your sexual relations.

The initial evaluation: both partners

Any investigation into the cause of infertility must involve both partners from the very start. The doctor should begin by interviewing both of you. Some aspects of the interview may be embarrassing, particularly when they deal with sexual histories and sexual practices. Certainly, these interviews can be conducted separately, and, of course, confidentially.

During this initial office visit, your doctor should discuss with you some of the emotional issues surrounding infertility, its diagnosis and treatment. (See Chapter 3 for more information on choosing the right doctor and Chapters 11, 12, and 13 for coping with the emotional side of infertility.)

Then the doctor should begin testing both the man and the woman. As you'll recall from Chapter 3, the woman will likely start with her OB/GYN. The man will probably be referred to a urologist or andrologist.

If the woman is the only one tested—as is all too often the case—or if the man is not tested for weeks or months, precious time, and probably money, may be wasted.

The diagnostic rationale

Finding a cause for infertility may not be straightforward. It's not like seeing a doctor for a broken arm. In fact, most times a couple seeks help because they only suspect they have a problem; once infertility is confirmed, then the task is to find its cause or causes and correct it or, sometimes, them. Sometimes them? Yes, because finding the solution to a moderately severe problem may be enough to achieve a pregnancy even if the partner still has an unresolved minor problem.

After an initial interview, your doctor will have some clues as to where the problem(s) may lie. Some avenues of investigation, or even treatment, might be obvious. If the man had a vasectomy in a first marriage but wants to have a child in his second, a vasectomy reversal might be the best option. If the woman is a marathon runner and hasn't had a menstrual period in years, getting her ovulating as soon as possible would be considered.

But in the infertility workup, causes are not usually so obvious. And, just because one, even obvious, cause is found doesn't mean that the diagnostic workup should stop there. So how does the doctor narrow the range of reasons for your infertility?

Your doctor will first look for the most likely reasons in your medical history, based on what is already known about the common causes of infertility. For example, a woman with a history of irregular, heavy menstrual periods would certainly undergo hormonal testing first. Because ovulatory and sperm problems are by far the most common causes of infertility, confirming ovulation and assessing sperm are mandatory early evaluations.

What about exploring the causes of infertility that occur with fairly equal frequency? Poor sperm and cervical mucus interaction, Fallopian tube or uterine problems, and even unexplained causes, all account for about the same percentage of infertility cases. The diagnostic principle here is to start with

Unofficially...
Ancient Egyptians believed that women could conceive through their mouths.

the least difficult and invasive tests—which are also usually the most revealing—and go on to the more difficult or invasive ones as needed.

Basically, your doctor is looking to determine four facts:

- Is the woman ovulating?
- Does the man have sufficient, healthy sperm?
- Can the sperm and the egg meet?
- Can a fertilized egg implant itself successfully?

Fortunately, answering these questions can sometimes be simple and won't involve expensive, difficult, or painful procedures. In fact, you perform some of these tests at home yourself.

The workup

The infertility workup is done systematically. That's not to say that it needs to be a drawn-out affair. Some parts can and should be done simultaneously. While the workup must be complete, you don't want to go through unnecessary, time-consuming, and expensive testing. So ask questions about what the tests will show. Some may be redundant or only give small, insignificant bits of information.

A basic, but thorough, infertility workup includes a *history, physical examination, routine office and laboratory tests*, and, only if necessary, more *specialized tests*.

Some aspects of the infertility workup are similar for any condition that brings you to a doctor and apply to both partners. And, as we said earlier, these early tests should be done in tandem. Some tests and timing may vary, however, if the woman is older than thirty-five years of age. For example, you and your doctor may want to move things along by scheduling several tests in one cycle or go quickly

Timesaver
Bring any earlier test results with you to the doctor. While some tests might be repeated because your fertility status can change over time, previous test results can be clues to what's going on now. Also, it's not unheard of for a new doctor to reinterpret test results and come to a different conclusion.

to more specialized tests, such as a laparoscopy (discussed in more detail later in this chapter). Some hormone tests, such as that for follicle stimulating hormone(FSH) test, are particularly helpful in older women hoping to conceive. (If you're over age thirty-five, remember: don't wait more than six months before seeking help if you suspect a fertility problem.)

History

The first step is to obtain a complete history: medical, surgical, and sexual.

Medical history

Bright Idea
Start thinking about the illnesses or habits you've had that might be impacting on your fertility. But don't feel guilty about anything! And ask your parents about childhood illnesses or injuries that might be affecting your fertility.

A complete medical history contains information not only about your personal health, but your family history, as well. In addition to questions about your overall health, the doctor will ask you specific questions about your current and previous fertility status. Because sexually transmitted diseases (STDs) are a major cause of infertility, your doctor should seek clues of present or past infection.

- *Current infertility.* How long have you been trying to conceive? What contraceptives have you used? And for how long? What infertility tests have you had? What treatments have you had?

- *Previous fertility.* If you're a woman, have you ever been pregnant? If you're a man, have you ever fathered a child?

Personal and family medical history

Your doctor will question you about diseases or disorders that "run in the family," as well as about your use of medications or drugs, and about lifestyle factors that may have an effect on your fertility.

- Do you have diabetes, hypertension, asthma, arthritis, ulcers, colitis, or thyroid disease? Have you had cancer? Were you treated with surgery, radiotherapy, or chemotherapy? Did your mother use DES (diethylstilbestrol)? If you're a man, were your testicles normal at birth, or did you have mumps as an adult? Is there a family history of genetic disorders such as cystic fibrosis, sickle-cell anemia, Tay-Sachs disease, muscular dystrophy, or hemophilia)?

■ What prescription and over-the-counter medicines do you take? Your doctor will ask you if you currently or have ever: Smoked? Used or abused alcohol? Taken illicit drugs? And, if so, how much do you use or have you used them?

■ What type of work do you do? What hobbies do you have? Have you ever come in contact with chemicals, pesticides, or radiation?

■ Have you had a sexually transmitted disease? If you're a woman, your doctor will also ask if you have ever had vague *genito-urinary* (abdominal, bladder, or vaginal) symptoms? The doctor may ask you about other risk factors for pelvic inflammatory disease (PID), such as number of past sexual partners. (See Chapter 2 for information on PID.)

Surgical history

If you're a woman, have you ever had an appendectomy or other abdominal or pelvic surgery? If you're a man, have you ever had surgery to correct a varicocele undescended testis (cryptorcidism), or hernia? Or any other groin, pelvis or bladder operation? (See Chapter 2 for more information about conditions and operations that might interfere with male fertility.)

Unofficially...
The earliest evidence of the link between occupation and infertility was noted by a French scientist in 1860 when he observed that wives of lead workers were less likely to become pregnant and more likely to miscarry when they did.

Sexual history

How frequently do you have intercourse? Do you have pain during sexual intercourse? What positions do you use? Do you achieve an orgasm? If you're a woman, do you douche, or use lubricants or feminine hygiene products? Does your partner's penis enter and penetrate your vagina? If you're a man, do you achieve and maintain an erection? Do you enter and penetrate your partner's vagina? Do you ejaculate into your partner's vagina?

Special questions about the woman's medical history

Besides current and previous fertility status, the doctor will ask the woman more in-depth questions about her gynecologic and obstetric history.

- *Gynecologic history.* When did you start menstruating? Are your menstrual periods regular? How long, heavy, or painful are they? Do you experience *mittelschmerz*—mild pain on one side of your abdomen near the time of ovulation? Do you have vaginal discharge? What gynecologic or urologic problems have you had? Have you had a *tubal ligation* (sterilization, sometimes called having your "tubes tied")?

- *Obstetrical history.* Have you ever been pregnant? When? How long did it take to get pregnant? Did you carry to term? Were there any complications? Did you breastfeed? For how long? Did you ever suffer a stillbirth? Have you had an abortion, either spontaneous or induced? Were there any complications?

Special questions about the man's medical history

The doctor will also have specific questions for the male partner to answer, specifically pertaining to his urologic history. Such questions will include: Have you ever had undescended testes (cryptorchidism), a varicocele, testicular injury, testicular torsion, or Klinefelter's syndrome? Have you ever had any infection such as epididymitis, prostatitis, or sexually transmitted diseases? Have you had a vasectomy? Have you been exposed to direct, excessive heat, radiation, or toxic chemicals? When did you enter puberty? (See Chapter 2 for more information on these and other causes of male infertility.)

The physical examination

Next comes the physical exam. Your doctor will be looking more for factors that might be contributing to infertility than for the cause of infertility itself. These can range from malnutrition to obesity, from renal to thyroid disease. Very importantly, the doctor will look for signs of hormone imbalance.

The physical examination of the woman: A complete physical exam of the woman includes vaginal, pelvic, and rectal examinations. Your doctor will look for obvious structural defects, such as the size, shape, or position of your reproductive organs, that might be interfering with conception. The exam might also suggest tumors, adhesions, or endometriosis, all risk factors for infertility. When inspecting the vaginal canal, the doctor will be looking for lesions and vaginal discharge, both of which might suggest an STD, and cervical tears, polyps or infection, any of which might interfere with sperm survival. The presence of excessive hair (hirsuitism) on the face, back and abdomen; acne; or obesity, might be clues to a hormonal imbalance that can interfere with reproduction.

The doctor might perform a routine Pap test to rule out cervical cancer or other abnormalities and take a sample of cervical secretions for culture to rule out infection. In particular, the doctor should be looking for that silent, prevalent organism

Unofficially...
One pizza worker was found to have impaired sperm development; standing in front of the hot pizza ovens every day brought his sperm count down.

Chlamydia trachomatis, which is a leading cause of infertility. (See Chapter 2 for more information about this and other sexually transmitted diseases.)

The physical examination of the man: The doctor—usually a urologist or andrologist—will examine the testes, penis, scrotum, and prostate, looking for any signs of structural deformities or infection. The doctor will also note the size and texture of the testes. In particular, the doctor will look for a varicocele, penile deformities (such as *hypospadias*), undescended testes, as well as examine the status of the epididymis and vas deferens. The doctor might also take a sample of urethral secretions or prostate fluid to be cultured to rule out infection.

Your doctor will look for outward signs of a hormone imbalance, such as enlarged breasts. In particular, the doctor will note your secondary sex characteristics, those that are regulated by testosterone, such as facial and body hair, and voice depth.

Routine office and laboratory tests

After the basic history and physical examination, your doctor will order routine office and laboratory tests designed to look more closely for specific female and male infertility factors. These tests are quite simple and will seek answers to the first two questions we mentioned earlier: Is the woman ovulating? Is the man producing enough healthy sperm?

Is the woman ovulating?

Because several hormones secreted in specific amounts and sequences regulate ovulation, testing for ovulation involves looking for signs that these hormones are present and measuring them at

Watch Out!
If you're told you have uterine fibroids and that's why you're not getting pregnant, you might consider a second opinion. Uterine fibroids are rarely the sole cause of infertility. If your tests don't show a distorted uterine cavity or tubal occlusion, and you don't feel a lot of pelvic pressure, it may be time check with someone else.

different times during the menstrual cycle. Keep in mind that these hormones are just markers, as doctors call them, for ovulation.

Your gynecologic history can give clues to your ovulatory status. A history of irregular or absent menstrual periods points strongly to an ovulatory problem. Here are the most common tests to help detect ovulation. They can be done at home.

A *basal body temperature (BBT) chart* detects when ovulation has likely taken place. Every morning before any activity, the woman takes her oral temperature and plots it on a chart. Over two to three months, the chart should show a pattern of slight temperature rise at mid-cycle (0.4° to 1.0°F), which plateaus until about the time of menstruation, as progesterone levels increase, indicating ovulation has taken place (this is called a *biphasic* pattern). If no temperature elevation is apparent (a *monophasic* pattern), further testing is needed. While the BBT is usually taken in the morning before getting out of bed, it can be taken last thing at night. The important thing is to take it at the same time each day.

The *urinary luteinizing hormone (LH) test* measures LH levels in the urine and pinpoints more accurately the LH surge that precedes ovulation. LH testing is performed daily for about four to five days at mid-cycle—which is about eleven days after the first day of a woman's period. It's a simple test that can be done in minutes at home—or actually anywhere. There are plenty of good kits on the market. At this point in the diagnostic process, it's probably a waste of money—and time—to go through daily blood drawing for hormone information that can be gained simply and far less expensively with an LH surge monitoring kit.

Unofficially...
A medical review compared four different ovulation tests. Transvaginal sonography was the most accurate, correctly finding ovulation 96 percent of the time. The next most accurate tests were serum LH levels (85 percent), BBT charting (77 percent), and chronologic dating based on the next menstrual cycle (65 percent).

Unlike BBT charting, the urinary LH test predicts ovulation. But both BBT charting and urinary LH measurements are used to help schedule other tests and procedures. They are also very helpful in scheduling sexual intercourse around a woman's most fertile days.

Even if you are ovulating, you may have a hormone imbalance that makes it impossible for a fertilized egg to implant itself in the endometrium. Only occurring in about three to five percent of women, this luteal phase defect is an important diagnostic consideration. (There will be more about tests for luteal phase defect later in this chapter.)

Your doctor might order additional tests to determine whether or not you're ovulating. These include blood tests to measure hormone levels, an endometrial biopsy, and vaginal ultrasound, all of which we'll look at more closely later.

The *cervical mucus test* is an easy, but vital, part of your infertility workup. Because cervical mucus changes consistency during the menstrual cycle, doctors can tell whether you're likely to be ovulating by examining cervical mucus characteristics. This is a test that either you or your doctor can do. Just before ovulation is anticipated, take a small sample of mucus from your vagina and cervical area. If it's watery, clear, and can be stretched pretty far (called *spinnbarkeit* factor), it's a good indication that ovulation is approaching. But this isn't a perfectly reliable test. Infection or prior cervical surgery can thicken mucus, making you think you don't ovulate. Also, some women produce good cervical mucus at the time of ovulation, but it stays in the cervical canal, unavailable for your inspection.

Is the man producing enough healthy sperm?

As we said earlier, the diagnostic workup of the man must begin immediately if infertility is a problem. Luckily, the most important diagnostic test for male factor infertility, the *semen analysis,* is simple, noninvasive, and certainly not painful. But some men may find it embarrassing. It answers the question: Are you producing sufficient healthy sperm?

Semen analysis evaluates the quantity and quality of sperm and seminal fluid. More than one analysis—usually three—may be done because semen quality varies and results can change over time. Semen analysis looks at several specific factors:

- *Volume* shows whether the ejaculate has the right amount and mix of substances needed to keep sperm alive and well.

- *Sperm count,* sometimes called sperm concentration or sperm density, shows whether enough sperm are being delivered with the ejaculate to make conception possible. (Sperm production can be normal but a blockage may cause sperm to be absent in the ejaculate.)

- *Sperm morphology* shows whether the sperm are shaped properly. There is another more sophisticated examination of sperm shape, called the *strict sperm morphology determination.* In this test, specially stained sperm are examined under a microscope. Precise measurements of sperm heads and tails are taken. Doctors pay particular attention to the width, length, and contours of heads and the lengths of the tails.

- *Sperm motility,* which may actually be more important than their number or concentration, shows whether the sperm can swim, and, more

Watch Out!
Not all technicians performing semen analysis are trained to interpret sperm morphology. Make sure your doctor uses a lab with specialized personnel.

importantly, whether they can swim fast and forward.

- *Sperm viscosity* shows whether semen—which is delivered into the vagina as thickish, jelly-like substance called coagulum—will finally liquefy. If it doesn't, it may affect sperm function.

- *White blood cells (WBC)*, if found in the semen, might point to an infection or inflammation. Sometimes WBC are difficult to distinguish from early sperm forms, so special stains or antibodies may be added to help.

Unofficially...
One-half of 1 percent of men were functionally sterile in 1938. Today, that percentage has increased fifteen-fold! Nearly 12 percent of men have sperm counts below 20 million/mL of semen and are therefore considered sterile.

A semen sample is usually collected by masturbation after two to three days of sexual abstinence. Some men find it difficult to masturbate on demand, at a doctor's office, or at all. Because of this, many facilities have special private rooms, replete with erotic literature and videos, and some encourage the partner to participate, to help the process along. It's important that the sample remain sterile, that it be kept at body temperature, and that it be analyzed within about an hour after collection.

If you need to bring a semen sample in for analysis, keep the container in a pocket closest to your body. Don't leave it on your dashboard to get baked in the sun or fried from the heater. And don't keep it near the air-conditioning vents either.

Don't waste good time on possible bad lab results. Ask your doctor about the lab doing your semen analysis, particularly if the lab is right there in your doctor's office. If it doesn't specialize in infertility assessment and handle several dozen analyses a month, it probably doesn't have the expertise to make accurate evaluations. Some doctors are using computer-assisted systems. While they

SEMEN ANALYSIS
(BASED ON AT LEAST TWO ANALYSES)

Parameter	Normal Range
Volume	2 to 5 mL (may be as low as 1 mL)
pH	7.4
Sperm count	50 to 200 million per mL (20 million is the lowest count that will allow pregnancy to occur naturally, without special treatment)
Sperm motility	50 to 80 percent progressive motility one hour after ejaculation
Sperm morphology	60 to 90 percent (may be as low as 30 percent)
Liquefaction time	10 to 20 minutes after ejaculation
Content	No or only minimal white cells or epithelial cells

have their place, they shouldn't be relied on solely, either. They require a well-trained and experienced person to make assessments. And the equipment needs to be calibrated. It's easy for the computer to count every little speck as a sperm, leading you to believe you have a higher sperm count than you really do. But it takes a skillful eye to evaluate other sperm characteristics, like how well formed they are. So, it's probably best if your doctor uses both methods to evaluate sperm quantity and quality.

More specialized tests may be needed if the results of the semen analyses show a problem. If sperm count is low, a man's blood testosterone FSH, and LH levels should be checked. *Urinalysis* is helpful in finding white blood cells, which may indicate infection. It will also spot sperm in the urine, which may be caused by retrograde ejaculation. (See Chapter 2 for more information on retrograde ejaculation.)

THE TIMING OF SOME BASIC INFERTILITY TESTS

Timing is everything, especially in infertility treatment. Here's a chart to help you see which tests are performed at the various points in the menstrual cycle. Remember, Day 1 is counted from the end of the last menstrual period:

Cycle Day(s)	Test	Why it's done at this time
Day 1 to Day 11	Hysterosalpingogram X-ray	This test evaluates the size and shape of the uterus prior to the changes that occur with ovulation. To be certain to avoid testing during ovulation, the test is usually scheduled toward the end of this part of the cycle (Days 10 or 11).
Day 12 to Day 15	Post-coital exam	This test checks to see if sperm live well in the cervical mucus. It is scheduled during the point in the cycle when cervical mucus conditions are likely to be most favorable to sperm.
Day 19 to Day 24	Progesterone blood test	This test checks the levels of progesterone being produced. Progesterone production increases at the time of ovulation, so this test is scheduled during that part of the cycle when its levels in the blood are highest.
Day 19 through Day 28	Endometrial biopsy	This test permits the evaluation of the tissue that lines the uterus to see if it can develop the structures necessary to support an implanted fetus. The test is done after ovulation, when the tissue lining the uterus is best developed.

Testing whether your sperm and egg can meet

The first test used to answer this question is rather simple. It's also one that you and your partner start at home—the doctor views the results in the office. It's the *postcoital (Sims-Huhner) test*. If the results of this test show a good number of moving sperm, other female factors might be explored with more specialized tests to determine what's interfering with fertilization. There may be a structural problem with your Fallopian tubes for example, that's preventing the egg and sperm from getting together.

The postcoital test is a very important test for cervical mucus problems that may be causing infertility. It gives some idea of how the sperm react in the lower female reproductive tract, as well as whether enough sperm are being deposited in the vagina. In fact, it has been considered for years what doctors call the gold standard for determining sperm survivability after intercourse. While an essential test, the postcoital test should never take the place of a complete semen analysis.

The postcoital test is performed just before ovulation, so BBT charting and urinary LH kits are helpful in scheduling this test. You should engage in sexual intercourse the night before, or on the morning of, the test. Don't douche! Don't use any lubricants! Don't use any vaginal medications, sprays, creams, or powders! The doctor will take a sample of the woman's cervical mucus—a painless procedure—and examine it under a microscope to see how many sperm are there and how well they're moving. There is some debate about exactly how long after intercourse the test should be done. Generally, about eight hours later is considered to

Bright Idea
The valve of the postcoital test for predicting future conception has come under serious question recently. Because information on the usefulness of this test is being gathered daily, it's a good idea to discuss how important its findings will be to your situation.

Bright idea
If you can't ejac-
ulate through
masturbation, try
using a nonsper-
micidal condom
during sexual
intercourse and
have that sample
tested. If you're
prohibited from
masturbating,
you might try
using a condom
with a pinhole in
it during sexual
intercourse. This
allows some
semen to enter
the woman's
vagina, where it
can then be
collected.

be the best time, but the range can be from three to twenty-four hours.

If too few moving sperm are seen under micro-scopic examination, it could mean that sperm production or delivery into the vagina is impaired. If the sperm are not moving, it could signal a prob-lem with the timing of the test, the cervical mucus itself or with antisperm antibodies. (The role, if any, of antisperm antibodies in infertility is, however, not as significant as once thought.) If the quality or quantity of the cervical mucus is poor, it may indi-cate a cervical abnormality or an infection.

Sometimes, your doctor will order this test a sec-ond time, but may set up your office visit sooner or later than he or she did for the first test. For exam-ple, if the test results are poor, you may be asked to come into the office sooner after sexual intercourse. If the test results are good, but you haven't con-ceived in a few months, you may be asked to come into the office for examination later after sexual intercourse.

Common hormone tests for the woman

In addition to your other tests, here are some blood tests your doctor might order:

- The *FSH (follicle stimulating hormone) test* helps distinguish ovarian failure from hypothalamic or pituitary problems. A basal measurement FSH on the first, second, or third day of the menstrual cycle is sometimes done when a woman is over thirty-five to see if she's experi-encing premature or early menopause. The results of the FSH test can give some clues to egg quality in general.

- The *LH (luteinizing hormone) test* will show if the hypothalamic/pituitary and gonadal systems are working properly. It can help distinguish between primary ovarian failure and gonadal stimulation.

■ *The estradiol (E₂)* test assesses how well the ovaries are functioning and whether egg follicles are maturing properly.

■ *Progesterone* testing will show whether ovulation has occurred and the corpus luteum is functioning normally. It's useful for determining that the uterine lining can receive a fertilized egg for implantation. Progesterone is another hormone that will give clues to a luteal phase defect.

■ *Prolactin* testing will show the presence or absence of prolactin. Abnormally high levels can interfere with or disrupt ovulation and/or progesterone production.

More specialized tests for the woman

The tests described below help evaluate the reproductive organs directly. Some, like the laparoscopy and hysteroscopy, are invasive and, usually, the final steps in the diagnostic workup. Remember, bring your partner or a friend with you to these tests to offer support and get you to and from the test site. Some of these tests—and the medications they give when you take them—may impair your ability for several hours.

■ *Hysterosalpingogram* is a special X-ray using a contrast dye to evaluate the size and shape of the uterus and determine if the Fallopian tubes are open. It's performed after a menstrual period, but before ovulation. Injected through the cervix, the dye fills the uterus and should flow freely into the Fallopian tubes. Your doctor

"
After putting off having a hysterosalpingogram for months, I finally had it done. Much to my surprise, they found that my tubes were slightly blocked. The doctor forced the dye through and the very next month I got pregnant through artificial insemination using my husband's sperm.
—Jane, a computer analyst.
"

will be looking for uterine scar tissue, polyps, fibroids, and deformities—conditions that prevent sperm and egg from meeting or embryo implantation, or induce a miscarriage.

This test can be, but is not always, very uncomfortable. So, you may want to ask for painkillers and muscle relaxants to ease the situation. Your doctor might also prescribe an antibiotic. You may have some discomfort, as well as discharge for a few hours after the test as dye is expelled. The uterus stretching as it fills with dye is the cause of the discomfort. If the tubes are blocked, pressure might build up and may also cause some pain. But the pressure from the injected dye might even open up small blockages.

- *Vaginal ultrasound* helps confirm ovulation. (Until a few years ago, pelvic ultrasounds, which were done externally, were used.) Because ultrasound works on the principle of sound waves bouncing off fluid-filled objects, if the follicle, which is a fluid-filled sac beneath the surface of the ovary, ripens, enlarges, and then collapses after an egg is released, the sonogram will detect it. Again, just because a deflated follicle is detected doesn't mean that it released an egg or had one in it to begin with. But a positive test result here plus positive results from LH surge and BBT charting raise the likelihood that you're ovulating.

A series of sonograms, starting after the LH surge and continuing until a collapsed follicle is detected, are taken to monitor ovulation. The bonus of this test is that it can provide information about endometrial lining thickness, which is an important factor in implantation. This information is important if your doctor suspects a luteal phase defect. Your doctor can also use the test to assess uterine and ovarian position and size and detect any cyst or pregnancy.

■ *Endometrial biopsy* is used to evaluate ovulation and luteal phase defect, in which the uterine lining can't support implantation. Comparing the biopsy to blood hormone test results can show if, indeed, ovulation *and* uterine preparation are normal.

Performed very quickly in the doctor's office, an endometrial biopsy is scheduled anywhere from the mid-luteal phase, or about Day 21 of the menstrual cycle, to just before a woman expects her menstrual period, that is, when progesterone-induced effects on the uterine lining are at their peak. A small piece of tissue is removed from the endometrium and examined under a microscope. A trained eye can tell if the tissue is responding properly to progesterone.

Two cautions: A pregnancy test must be done before the biopsy, and you might have some mild discomfort during and after the test or some mild spotting after, so ask for some analgesics.

■ *Laparoscopy* is an invasive, usually outpatient, procedure ideally done after menstrual flow is done but before ovulation, with the patient under general anesthesia. It allows the doctor to look directly at the Fallopian tubes, ovaries, and the outside of the uterus through a telescopic instrument inserted through a small incision in or near the navel. (Sometimes other small cuts are made to allow a better look at the pelvic organs.) Your doctor will check for

Timesaver
If you're having a diagnostic laparoscopy or hysteroscopy, discuss with your doctor correcting any problem found right then and there. It will save the time, expense, and discomfort of undergoing the procedure a second time. But be certain the doctor performing the test is qualified to correct any problems.

endometriosis, adhesions, fibroids, and ovarian cysts. The doctor can also inject a solution through the cervix and uterus to see if the Fallopian tubes are open. You may have some pain, stiffness, and soreness for a day or two after the procedure.

- *Hysteroscopy* is also an invasive, usually outpatient procedure, scheduled just after a woman's menstrual period, and done under general or local anesthesia. A telescopic instrument is inserted through the dilated cervix into the lower end of the uterus. Gas or a clear fluid is injected into the uterus so that the uterine cavity expands and blood and mucus are cleared. Your doctor will be looking inside the uterus for fibroids, polyps, scarring, and congenital deformities.

Note! ➡
Laparoscopy.

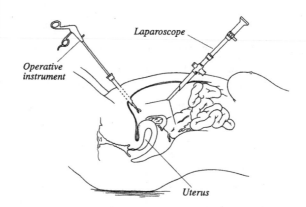

More specialized tests for men

The advent of high-tech procedures, such as the assisted reproductive technologies (ARTs) that we will examine in depth in Chapters 7 and 8, have led to the declining use of several diagnostic tests for male-factor infertility. But, it's important that the male partner undergo urologic evaluation to ensure that correctable causes of multi-factor infertility are not overlooked and that the infertility is not an indication of some significant underlying health problem.

The sperm agglutination test is a laboratory test in which sperm are looked at under the microscope to see if they clump together. Clumping prevents sperm from swimming through cervical mucus and attaching to an egg. Antisperm antibodies or an infection can cause sperm agglutination. (See Chapter 2 for more information about antisperm antibodies.) As we noted earlier, it's unclear how much, if any, antisperm antibodies interfere with fertility. Current data has raised questions about the usefulness of this test, so it's being used less and less frequently.

The *hamster penetration assay* or *sperm penetration assay (SPA)* are tests that were used more often in years past than they are today. They served to discover whether sperm are actually capable of penetrating deep inside an egg and fertilizing it. In this laboratory test, sperm are put near hamster eggs that have been specially stripped of their outermost layer, the zona pellucida, so that human sperm can penetrate, but not fertilize, them. (It's the zona pellucida that protects eggs produced by one species from being fertilized with sperm from other species.) If too few sperm penetrate too few hamster eggs, it may indicate that the sperm are unable to penetrate a woman's egg. Because the results may not correlate with fertility, many fertility specialists no longer use them.

The *hemizona assay* is a more specialized test of sperm function. This test uses discarded, nonusable human eggs with their zona pellucida intact. The eggs are cut in half to see if the man's sperm, and sperm from a control sample of sperm, can pierce through the outermost protective layer of the egg.

Some centers will run the two tests at the same time to give a very clear picture of how well the man's sperm can fertilize an egg. These tests may be used when infertility is unexplained and in preparation for assisted reproductive technologies. (See Chapter 7, on assisted reproductive technologies, for more information about these and other tests.)

If routine laboratory test results are inconclusive or don't point to a specific problem, more sophisticated testing might be needed. Some evaluate sperm quality, some sperm production. Others assess sperm transport. Here are a few of the tests that might be ordered and why:

- The *acrosome reaction test* determines whether sperm heads can actually undergo the chemical changes needed to dissolve an egg's tough outer shell and penetrate it.

- *The hypo-osmotic swelling test* is sometimes used to help predict whether sperm can fertilize an egg. Normal sperm tails will swell when put into a special sugar and salt solution. Dead or poorly functioning sperm membranes don't seem to possess that characteristic.

- *Testicular biopsy* is done to determine how well sperm are being produced. In this test, a very small piece of tissue taken from the *seminiferous tubules* and surrounding areas (*interstitial tissue*) is examined under a microscope for signs of abnormal sperm production.

- *Hormone tests* are sometimes as important in evaluating male factor infertility as they are for female factor infertility. Blood samples are taken and assessed for FSH and LH, which are both critical for sperm development and maintaining testosterone levels. Elevated prolactin levels may indicate low testosterone levels and even impotence.

- *The vasography,* which is an X-ray of the vas deferens, is used to find a blockage or leakage of sperm.

- *High-resolution scrotal ultrasonography* and *venography* are tests to find varicoceles in the testicles too small to be felt during physical examination.

- *Ultrasonography* is used to find damages or blockages in the male reproductive tract, including the prostate, seminal vesicles, and ejaculatory ducts.

Watch Out!
Because sperm quality can vary over time—in fact, even a slight fever will change the results of a semen analysis—make sure the doctor orders two or three analyses over a two- to six-month period.

Taking the steps to diagnosing infertility

After reading this chapter, you've probably saved yourself considerable time because you've had a chance to think about some of the questions your doctor will be asking and, if need be, researched some of the answers before seeing your doctor.

Here are just a few other questions that may help you and your partner begin to explore where your diagnostic journey takes you:

- Do we understand why these tests are being done? Are we prepared to handle the results?

- How do we feel about some of the personal questions about our sex lives that we'll be asked?

- Can we afford this?

- How much time will this take? Do we have time to wait?

- Do our personal or religious beliefs prevent either of us from pursuing this?

Just the facts

- Infertility diagnosis should involve both partners being evaluated simultaneously.

- Ask your doctor why any test is being performed, if it is necessary, and if it will hurt. And keep asking until you fully understand the answers.

- Sexually transmitted diseases, in particular chlamydial infection and gonorrhea, contracted years ago may be hampering fertility today.

- When undergoing laparoscopy, ask your doctor if any abnormality can be fixed during that procedure.

- Understand the risk of any test, especially one that involves surgery.

- Two to three semen analyses should be performed before a baseline level is determined.

Finding the Right Treatment

GET THE SCOOP ON...
Fertility drugs ▪ Avoiding side effects ▪
Genetic engineering ▪ Semen collection

PART III

Fertility Drugs and Other Noninvasive Treatments

Chapter 5

Once you've found a qualified doctor with whom you and your partner are comfortable and you've gone through a thorough diagnostic evaluation, you'll probably have a good idea of what's causing your problem. Unless you and your partner have conditions that clearly call for surgery, infertility treatment usually begins with nonsurgical or noninvasive measures—often this means fertility drugs.

In fact, fertility drugs are a mainstay of infertility treatment. Certainly, you'll be given fertility drugs if you have obvious ovulatory dysfunction. It's estimated that infertility due to hormonal problems can be treated successfully with *ovulation induction* (as treatment with fertility drugs is called) in as many as 75 percent of all cases. This figure approaches the percentage rate of conception in the normal population.

101

How age affects fertility drug treatment

As a woman ages, her ovaries become more resistant to hormonal stimulation, either by infertility treatment or by the body itself, producing fewer follicles and eventually causing abnormally elevated serum FSH levels. Also, ovarian production of estrogen and progesterone declines, sometimes causing irregular menstrual cycles or even making the uterus less able to accept a pregnancy. Finally, fertilized oocytes are less likely to develop successfully into live births.

It's been known for years that a woman's chances of getting pregnant, carrying a pregnancy to term, and delivering a healthy, normal baby diminish steadily as she ages. Today, doctors are realizing that this reduced reproductive ability is due largely to poor egg quality.

Older women given traditional fertility drug regimens don't always get good results. New combinations are becoming available to help improve egg production in women over forty. And pregnancy rates in women who have no other infertility problems and who are given injectable fertility drugs are at least as high as those in women who ovulate normally. Unfortunately, as we discussed in Chapter 1, older women have a higher miscarriage rate.

Fertility drugs for all types of infertility

You may be surprised to learn that fertility drugs, many of which are actual hormones, are used to treat some types of male factor infertility, as well. Also, in cases of male factor infertility, the female partner is sometimes given fertility drugs to ensure *that* she ovulates and to pinpoint the time *when* she ovulates. With these assurances, procedures such as *therapeutic insemination* (*TI*, sometimes called *artificial insemination,* or *AI*) can be carried out at the woman's most fertile time. Therapeutic insemination is another important nonsurgical infertility treatment, which we will discuss in more detail later in this chapter.

If you're an older woman, or the cause of your infertility is not identified, fertility drugs are often prescribed to help boost the quality of your ovulations. In addition, sometimes both partners may be subfertile. In these cases, fertility drugs may be just the solution needed to compensate for subtle fertility shortcomings. (But make sure that every step is taken to address poor sperm quantity or quality as well if male factor infertility is also a problem.)

Finally, fertility drugs are an integral part of assisted reproductive technologies (ARTs). Here they're used to increase the number of eggs produced and to schedule these high tech procedures. (See Chapters 7 and 8 for more information on ARTs.)

It's likely, then, that at some point in your infertility treatment, fertility drugs may be an option for you. So it makes sense for anyone facing infertility treatment to understand these drugs and what they can do for you. But, of course, fertility drugs are not the only noninvasive infertility treatment available. In this chapter, we'll look at several others, as well.

The basics of hormonal control

Before we get started on the treatments themselves, however, a quick review of key points in the hormonal orchestration needed for ovulation, fertilization, and implantation is in order. (For a more detailed description of the female reproductive system, including hormonal control, see Chapter 1.)

Here are the steps involved in the natural, untreated menstrual cycle:

1. The hypothalamus releases *gonadotropin-releasing hormone (GnRH)* in a series of discrete, pulsed bursts that increase in the later part of the menstrual cycle.

2. The pituitary gland, in response to the GnRH signal, releases *follicle stimulating hormone (FSH)* and *luteinizing hormone (LH)*. It's primarily FSH that stimulates follicles to mature. (Anywhere from twenty to several hundred eggs and their follicles emerge from a resting state in the ovaries during each cycle. But only one or two become dominant and eventually release their eggs.)

3. Follicles, as they mature, release their own set of hormones, primarily estradiol, a type of estrogen.

4. In response to estrogen, the pituitary gland releases less and less FSH. If all goes correctly, only enough hormones, in particular FSH, are produced to keep the best follicles maturing.

5. At mid-cycle, the follicle fully matures or ripens. LH levels increase, or surge, to stimulate the follicle to ovulate, that is, release its egg.

6. The empty follicle becomes the *corpus luteum*, a hormone-producing structure, and begins releasing progesterone, which helps the endometrium become receptive to implantation of a fertilized egg.

Bright Idea
To lessen the pain, swelling, or irritation associated with a hormone injection, alternate injection sites: give it once in one buttock, next time in the front of the thigh, next in the other buttock, and then in the other thigh.

Ovulatory dysfunction and fertility drugs

Ovulatory dysfunction is by far the most common cause of female factor infertility, accounting for one-quarter to one-third of all infertility cases. Ovulatory dysfunction is the failure of the ovaries to produce or release an egg regularly, usually because of a hormonal imbalance. The aim of ovulation induction using fertility drugs is to bring these hormones back into line so that an egg is regularly available for fertilization each cycle.

What fertility drugs treat

Fertility drugs are helpful to treat a variety of ovulatory disorders, including:

- Failure to ovulate (*anovulation*)
- Infrequent ovulation (*oligo-ovulation*)
- Erratically occurring periods
- Luteal phase defects, both short and long
- Absence of menstruation (*amenorrhea*)

First, the aim of fertility drugs for these problems and for the procedures we'll discuss later in this chapter is to stimulate the production of a limited number of eggs—one or two of them. This is sometimes called *controlled ovarian hyperstimulation*. Obviously, having eggs available is critical for pregnancy to occur.

Second, as we said earlier, fertility drugs help to regulate the ovulatory cycle. This allows you to time sexual intercourse and schedule a TI.

Third, fertility drugs play a vital role in *assisted reproductive technologies (ART)*, as well. In ART, fertility drugs are used to increase the number of viable eggs per cycle—sometimes to more than a dozen—with the hope of improving the chances of fertilization and implantation. (Usually only two or three, but on occassion more embryos are transferred, however, in ART. The remaining eggs or embryos can be cryopreserved for future transfer attempts, if desired. See Chapter 7 for a full discussion of ART.)

Last, hormones are often given to prepare the uterus for embryo implantation, for ART procedures, particularly when using third-party reproductive procedures involving donor embryos. See Chapter 10 for third-party reproduction.

What to remember about fertility drug treatment

There are some particulars to remember when you're considering taking fertility drugs. Keep in mind that ovulation induction is a custom-tailored therapy. That's one reason why you need to be under the care of a specialist—usually a reproductive endocrinologist—who understands how to use these drugs appropriately. Several factors determine what fertility drug or drugs you're given and how much of them you should take.

First, your doctor will determine which hormone or hormones are malfunctioning. Depending on your hormonal profile, you may be prescribed one or more fertility drugs. And, depending on your clinical picture, treatment can take several directions. One strategy may be to replace a missing hormone. Another is to prescribe one hormone that will stimulate the release of the missing one. Other, strategies include giving low doses of a drug for a prolonged period and giving high doses for a short time.

Second, it's important to remember that not every treatment cycle ends with a viable and available egg. Sometimes, the hormonal juggling takes time to refine. It could be several months before a good-quality ovulation occurs. Remember, too, that a treatment cycle might have to be abandoned if your ovaries look ready to release too many eggs.

This would increase the risk of multiple pregnancy. Of course, if you're planning an ART procedure the goal of ovulation induction is to have many good-quality eggs available for retrieval and fertilization. But this is not the aim of ovulation induction when sexual intercourse or TI is the mechanism for fertilization.

Third, be advised that fertility drugs are not to be taken for months on end. Many of these agents are quite powerful. In general, if they don't work within a few months—ideally, within six—you must start looking at other treatments and reevaluate your treatment goals.

Other considerations to keep in mind:

- Fertility drugs require careful monitoring. The oral ones, such as clomiphene citrate, require minimal monitoring. But the injectable ones, containing FSH (either alone or in conjunction with LH), need intense monitoring. Your doctor must be able to gauge your response to therapy and calculate how much of a drug or drugs you need at a particular time. This part of the hormonal balancing act is guided by the results of tests you'll take throughout your treatment cycle. (See the following two sections for more information about specific monitoring of ovulation induction.)

- Fertility drugs can throw your emotions off balance. These drugs can exaggerate the mood swings many women experience during their menstrual cycles. These PMS-like symptoms can wreak havoc with your emotional state. The mood swings are in addition to the anticipation and disappointments associated with any fertility treatment.

Moneysaver
If you're traveling while taking fertility drugs that need refrigeration, get a hotel room with a small refrigerator. It's cheaper than having to throw away spoiled medicine. And don't forget to ask about how to store medicine during airplane flights.

▪ Fertility drugs do carry some risks—another reason for careful monitoring. Of course, with today's improved drug regimens and advanced monitoring techniques, by and large the use of fertility drugs is very safe when prescribed and monitored by qualified doctors.

Why monitoring is needed

It's critical that you be monitored carefully for the effects these drugs are having on your ovarian system. Monitoring is done for several reasons:

▪ To assess your response to the fertility drugs and to make adjustments as needed.

▪ To be certain that too many eggs are not being produced in any one cycle. Because fertility drugs can cause more than one egg to be produced, the likelihood of multiple pregnancies increases. With multiple gestation come inherent risks: multiple births, premature delivery, low-birth weight babies, and miscarriage. Certainly, these are issues for you, your partner, and your doctor to discuss. The majority of pregnancies—more than 75 percent—following ovulation induction are singletons, about 20 percent are twins. Far fewer are triplets or more.

▪ To determine when ovulation occurs. This allows doctors to maximize the chance of fertilization, whether done through sexual intercourse, therapeutic insemination, or assisted reproductive technology.

▪ To avoid *ovarian hyperstimulation syndrome (OHSS)*, a potentially serious or even life-threatening syndrome. As its name implies, OHSS results when the ovaries are overstimulated to produce eggs. The ovaries may enlarge and fluid may accumulate in the abdomen.

Ovarian Hyperstimulation Syndrome (OHSS)

Up to 10 percent of women undergoing ovulation induction may develop mild OHSS, but less than 1 percent get so serious a case that they require hospitalization. In fact, the risk of OHSS is rare with some fertility drugs, such as clomiphene citrate. Women with *polycystic ovarian disease (PCOD)*, sometimes called *Stein-Leventhal syndrome* or *hyperandrogenism*, are at particular risk for OHSS. They tend to develop many small follicles, rather than a few large ones, which increases the chances of OHSS.

The early warning signs of OHSS include: pelvic pain, nausea, vomiting, weight gain, and reduced urine output. In more serious cases, fluid can accumulate in the lungs, causing difficulty breathing. In extreme but rare cases, an ovary can rupture. OHSS can also lead to blood clots in the veins and lungs, as well as stroke.

Onset can be sudden and usually occurs about one week after ovulation or about seven to ten days after FSH treatment. If you're on FSH-containing regimens, you'll need to be monitored for at least two weeks after completing therapy.

How ovulation induction is monitored

When you're taking fertility drugs you'll be undergoing tests periodically throughout your treatment cycle. The most critical tests are:

- Ultrasound, which is used to detect if and how many follicles are developing and to detect their release.

- Blood tests, which measure hormone levels throughout your treatment cycle. Your doctor will use the test results to determine any dosage adjustments needed.

In addition to these important tests, your doctor will examine you for signs of possible side effects of the medication. (There will be more information on the risks of fertility drugs later in this chapter.) Your doctor may also perform a postcoital test to evaluate cervical mucus quality. The postcoital test is used if you're taking hormones that have anti-estrogen properties, which can thicken your cervical mucus, making it less amenable to sperm movement.

Your doctor may also have you chart your basal body temperature (BBT) and use ovulation kits to help assess the way you're responding to oral drugs. (See Chapter 2 for more information on BBT and ovulation kits.)

Now that you've got a pretty good idea what fertility drugs are supposed to do, how your doctor will monitor your response to them, and what pitfalls are involved, we'll give you some specific questions to ask your doctor before you start treatment.

Just as we said in Chapter 4 concerning diagnostic tests, you should feel free to ask questions. Always ask, "What does this drug do?" "What are its side effects?" "How long do I have to be on it?" "When can I expect to see results?" "What are its risks?" "What monitoring will I need while taking these drugs?"

Be sure to ask your doctor if you need to restrict any activities while taking the drugs. And, get written instructions for the medicines you are prescribed. This includes information about storing, handling, and, particularly, administering the drugs. Many of these drugs must be mixed and given by injection—a task that not everyone can or wants to do alone.

The more you know about these drugs the better prepared you'll be for some of the physical and

emotional ups and downs that they can cause, as
well as the ups and downs of success or failure during each treatment cycle.

A guide to fertility drugs

To make this section easier to read, we've provided
a table and a detailed list of the common fertility
drugs, using their generic or chemical names, fol-
lowed by their brand names. For example,
clomiphene citrate, a widely prescribed fertility drug, is
a generic name. It's available under the brand
names SEROPHENE or CLOMID.

One thing to keep in mind is that most fertility
drugs are actually the hormones themselves so they
really don't have bona fide generic names. *Human
menopausal gonadotropin (hMG)* is the hormone
name and that's what's given. Table 5.1, appearing
later in this chapter, should help guide you through
the alphabet soup of hormones and fertility drugs.

Listed after the generic and brand names are
their routes of administration, that is, how the drugs
are given. You take most of these drugs by injection.
In general, the older drug formulations are given
intramuscularly (IM), that is, by injection deep into
the muscle tissue using a very thick needle. You
probably can't give these injections to yourself so
you'll need to enlist the help of your partner or
designated assistant.

Many of the newer drug formulations—
particularly those developed through genetic
engineering—are injected subcutaneously (SC),
that is, under the skin using small, thin needles.
These are much easier to give to yourself. Some fertility drugs are taken orally. And, occasionally, a
drug may be given in a nasal spray.

Bright Idea
If your partner
travels a lot,
recruit a back-up
person to give
you your
injections.

Next comes a description of what doctors call the drug's mechanism of action—in other words, how it works. We'll then describe the drug's uses and tell you what to expect. As we said earlier, injectable fertility drugs require careful monitoring throughout your treatment cycle. We've already discussed some of the tests (for example, lab assessments, ultrasound exams, physical exams, and postcoital tests) you'll likely undergo and why. We'll just list the tests that are likely to be performed. You can refer back to the section on drug monitoring for the rationale behind these tests.

Finally, we'll list side effects and risks. We're not going to go into dosages because that really depends on your hormone levels are at a particular time. The dosage will likely be changed several times during your treatment. Suffice it to say that you should always ask how much of a drug you should be taking and ask again whenever the dosage is changed.

We're also not going to give you specifics on how long to be on any particular drug(s); that's a determination only you and your doctor can make. We'll just leave you with the caveat that you should not be taking any of these drugs for more than several months.

Clomiphene citrate

This is one of the most useful drugs available to treat female factor infertility. It's certainly one of the oldest and least expensive.

Brand names: CLOMID, SEROPHENE
Route of adminstration: Orally.
How it works: Clomiphene citrate is an anti-estrogen, that is, it blocks estrogen receptors in the hypothalamus, causing it to think you have an estrogen deficiency. As a result the hypothalamus signals the

TABLE 5.1: FERTILITY DRUGS:
FACTS AND DESCRIPTIONS

Generic/Chemical Name	Brand Name	How It's Given
Clomiphene Citrate	Serophene®, Clomid®	Tablet
Human menopausal gonadotropin (hMG)	Pergonal®, Humegon™, Repronex™	Injection (IM) Injection (IM) Injection (IM)
Follicle stimulating hormone (FSH)	Metrodin®, Follistim™,	Injection (IM) Injection (IM or SC)
	Gonal-F®, Fertinex™	Injection (SC) Injection (SC)
Human chorionic gonadotropin (hCG)	Pregnyl®, Profasi®, A.P.L.®	Injection (IM) Injection (IM) Injection (IM)
Bromocriptine suppository	Parlodel®	Tablets, Vaginal suppository
Gonadotropin-releasing hormone (GnRH)	Factrel®,	Injection (IM or SC)
	Lutrepulse®	Pump
Gonadotropin-release hormone agonists Leuprolide acetate, nafarelin acetate, and goserelin acetate	Lupron®, Synarel®, Zoladex®	Injection (IM or SC) Nasal spray Skin implants
IM = intramuscular		SC = Subcutaneous

pituitary gland to secrete more FSH and LH. The rising FSH levels stimulate follicle development. As the follicle develops, it secretes estrogen on its own. After therapy is stopped, the hypothalamus senses the high estrogen levels and signals the pituitary to begin the LH surge and egg release. If you don't get your periods you'll first be given a progesterone-like drug to produce menses.

Uses: To stimulate ovulation if you have infrequent periods, long cycles, or luteal phase defect. (Sometimes, luteal phase defect can be a side effect of clomiphene citrate therapy.) If you don't have

Moneysaver
If you're putting
some infertility
treatments or
prescriptions on
credit cards, use
ones that give
incentives, like
frequent flier
miles. And use
those bonus
miles to escape
for awhile.

any periods, you shouldn't be taking clomiphene citrate until pregnancy is ruled out.

What to expect: Clomiphene citrate is typically taken daily for five consecutive days, starting several days after your menstrual period begins. Exactly when to begin treatment depends on your particular hormone profile. If you haven't gotten your period in a while, your doctor might prescribe a *progestin,* usually *medroxyprogesterone* (PROVERA, NORLUTATE) or give you a shot of progesterone to bring on a period. If clomiphene works, you should ovulate about a week after your last pill.

Tests you'll take: Your doctor will probably order a postcoital test to be certain the drug's not thickening your cervical mucus. If it is, your doctor may prescribe estrogen or prednisone following clomiphene citrate therapy to help normalize cervical mucus consistency. If that doesn't work, *intrauterine insemination,* a procedure we'll discuss in more detail later, or other hormones (LH or FSH) are options.

You may have to chart your BBT and use ovulation predictor kits. You might undergo a pelvic exam to see how you're responding to the drug. To make certain you aren't developing any ovarian cysts, you might undergo a pelvic exam or ultrasound test before another treatment cycle is begun. Unless you have a complex case or an ART is planned, blood tests and ultrasound monitoring are rarely used if the ovulation tests are positive.

The majority of pregnancies occur in the first three cycles of clomiphene citrate use in women who don't ovulate regularly. The number falls dramatically after the first six cycles.

Risks: There's less of a risk of multiple gestation with clomiphene citrate than with other fertility drugs. The chance for twins is about 10 percent; the likelihood of more than two babies is 1 percent. Overstimulation of the ovaries may cause ovarian cysts, which is the reason a pelvic exam should be performed before each new cycle is begun. Severe hyperstimulation is rare with this drug.

Side effects: Side effects are dose dependent, which means the more of the drug you take, the more likely and worse the side effects. You may experience hot flushes, and mood swings on the days you take your pills, while depression, nausea, and breast tenderness may occur later in the cycle. If you develop severe headaches or vision problems, stop taking your medication and call your doctor.

Human chorionic gonadotropin (hCG)

Brand names: PROFASI, PREGNYL, A.P.L.

Route of administration: IM Injection.

How it works: hCG is similar chemically to LH, and, therefore, produces an LH surge, which causes a follicle to release an egg.

Uses: Most women undergoing ovulation induction will not release eggs spontaneously. Although hCG does what LH does, it has a longer duration of action than LH and is cheaper and easier to use.

If you're just undergoing standard ovulation induction—not superovulation induction in preparation for an ART—hCG isn't given if too many follicles seem to be developing. That exposes you to too great a risk of multiple pregnancies.

Side effects: Lower abdominal tenderness, redness or tenderness at injection site, hot flashes.

Human menopausal gonadotropin (hMG), FSH, and LH combined in equal amounts

Brand names: PERGONAL, HUMEGON, REPRONEX

Route of administration: IM injection.

How it works: Stimulates ovaries (*gonads*) directly to produce several eggs in one cycle.

Uses: hMG is the most potent fertility drug available. If clomiphene citrate hasn't worked, particularly if you need more FSH, you may be given hMG. It will raise FSH levels substantially and keep them elevated for longer periods than clomiphene citrate. hMG is also useful in women who do not menstruate. And, like clomiphene citrate, it's sometimes given if you're planning an ART procedure.

What to expect: Injections are usually given daily for seven to twelve days, starting on Day 2, 3, or 4 of the menstrual period. Because hMG is very potent, follicle development is monitored closely by ultrasound and blood estrogen levels. If your ovaries aren't responding, the dose may be increased. Once one or two large follicles are seen and estrogen levels are appropriate, an injection of hCG is given to stimulate their release. (Occasionally, women taking hMG will release eggs on their own.) If too many developing eggs are detected, the hCG injection is withheld.

Unlike clomiphene citrate, hCG has no anti-estrogen effects, so it won't adversely affect cervical mucus quality. In fact, it may have the opposite effect—it may make it easier for sperm to reach the cervix.

Risks: Because hMG is so potent, the risk of multiple pregnancy is higher than for clomiphene citrate. Ectopic pregnancy, spontaneous abortions, and premature deliveries may be increased in a woman taking hMG, too.

Side effects: Breast tenderness; pain, rash, swelling or rash at the injection site; abdominal bloating or pain; mood swings. The most serious side effect is

OHSS. (See the discussion of OHSS earlier in this chapter.)

Follicle stimulating hormone (FSH)

Brand names: METRODIN, FOLLISTIM, GONAL-F, FERTINEX

Route of administration: Injection. (METRODIN: IM; FOLLISTIM: IM or SC; GONAL-F and FERTINEX: SC.)

How it works: Stimulates follicle growth directly.

Uses: FSH is usually given when clomiphene hasn't worked. Because these drugs contain FSH with very little LH, they're also helpful when used in women with *polycystic ovarian syndrome*, a common ovulatory disorder in which LH levels are high, but FSH levels are low or normal.

What to expect: FSH is usually given daily for about a week or so early in the cycle. Ovulation usually happens within one to two weeks of treatment.

Like women undergoing treatment with hCG, women taking FSH are monitored with ultrasound and blood estrogen tests and receive an injection of hCG to stimulate follicle release. (Sometimes women given FSH will release eggs on their own.)

Risks: Similar to those for hMG.

Side Effects: Similar to those for hMG.

Bromocriptine

Brand name: PARLODEL

Route of administration: Orally or via vaginal suppository.

How it works: Reduces pituitary gland secretion of prolactin.

Uses: Bromocriptine is useful in women with high prolactin levels, which inhibits FSH and LH release.

What to expect: Bromocriptine is used several times daily until prolactin levels return to normal.

Treatment is quite successful, although some women do need to take clomiphene citrate or hMG, as well.

Risks: Bromocriptine does not increase the risk of multiple pregnancies.

Side effects: Nausea, vomiting, nasal congestion, headache, dizziness, fainting, decreased blood pressure. (Many of these side effects can be alleviated by using the vaginal suppository form of the drug. Side effects usually stop within 7 to 10 days.)

Gonadotropin-releasing hormone (GnRH)

Brand name: FACTREL, LUTREPULSE

Route of administration: Injection (IM or SC), or by intravenous (IV) infusion or pump.

How it works: Replaces missing GnRH and directly stimulates the pituitary to release FSH and LH.

Uses: Given to women who have failed to ovulate while taking clomiphene acetate or hMG. It's also used if you have specific types of hormonal problems, such as PCOD and luteal phase defect.

What to expect: A few follicles are produced. It is given during the luteal phase.

Risks: Slight chance of multiple births and mild OHSS.

Side effects: Nausea and headache; pain, swelling, and occasionally infection at the injection site.

GnRH agonists

Brand names: LUPRON (leuprolide acetate), SYNAREL (nafarelin acetate), ZOLADEX (goserelin acetate)

Route of administration: LUPRON via IM or SC injection; SYNAREL (nafarelin acetate) via nasal spray; ZOLADEX (goserelin acetate) via skin implants.

How it works: Causes LH and FSH release from the pituitary, eventually exhausting its supply.

Unofficially... Ancient Greeks believed that both men and women secreted semen. A pregnancy was the result of a couple's combined semen remaining in the woman.

Uses: GnRH agonists allow precise ovulation induction by suppressing normal ovarian function. By wiping out any natural GnRH production, they provide a hormonal "clean slate" on which to prescribe the exact amounts of FSH and LH needed without worrying about how much your body's on it's own.

GnRH agonists have been particularly helpful for women planning ART procedures. They have reduced the number of cancelled ART treatment cycles because of poor response to fertility drugs or premature ovulation. Long-acting GnRH agonists are sometimes given to women with polycystic ovarian disease (PCOD), endometriosis, and uterine fibroids.

What to expect: GnRH agonists can be given to suppress endometriosis, and shrink fibroids and PCOD cysts.

Side Effects: Very similar to those seen in menopausal women including hot flashes, headaches, mood swings, insomnia, vaginal dryness, vaginal dryness leading to painful intercourse, reduced breast size, and bone loss.

Risks: Disruption of menstrual cycle.

Other common nonsurgical treatments for male or female infertility

One of the most common, oldest, simplest, and successful, treatments available to overcome several male, as well as female infertility problems is *therapeutic,* sometimes called *artificial, insemination (TI or AI)* using the husband's or donor sperm.

Therapeutic (artificial) insemination by any name

For decades, these procedures were called *artificial inseminations,* AI for short. In more recent years, they have been known as *therapeutic inseminations,* TI

Watch Out!
An optimal semen specimen is obtained when the man refrains from ejaculation for at least forty-eight hours prior to providing a specimen. But don't abstain for more than five to seven days. Sperm quality decreases with prolonged storage in the body.

for short. To confuse matters further, when the woman was artificially inseminated with her husband's sperm, the procedure was called AIH—the "H" standing for "husband." When sperm from a donor was used, the procedures were referred to as "AID," the "D" standing for "donor." With the growing and legitimate concern of contracting HIV, the virus that causes AIDS, from donor sperm, these procedures are usually now referred to as *TI-H* and *TI-D*. (We'll discuss donor sperm in greater detail in Chapter 8.)

Whether using the sperm from the husband or a donor, the goal is to place a large number of sperm close to the point of fertilization. Sometimes the procedure is done several times during ovulation to optimize the chance of fertilization.

Once it's been determined that the woman doesn't have problems that would seriously impede fertilization, such as damaged Fallopian tubes or implantation problems, TI is quite useful. What's critical is that she be ovulating. In fact, TI is often performed in conjunction with ovulation induction. (See the specific information about the goals of ovulation induction, earlier in this chapter.)

TI is useful in men with retrograde ejaculation, premature or delayed ejaculation, or structural defects that prevent sperm from being deposited in the vagina. It's also helpful in bypassing the cervix when the woman's cervical mucus is poor or she produces antisperm antibodies. TI is often used in couples with unexplained infertility. (See Chapter 2 for more information about the causes of male and female infertility.) There are two TI techniques: *intracervical insemination* (ICI) and *intrauterine insemination* (IUI).

■ In ICI, the male produces a semen specimen, typically through masturbation. (Other techniques to collect sperm are discussed at the end of this chapter.) If donor sperm are used, a frozen specimen collected at least six months earlier is thawed and used. The specimen is placed in the cervix using a syringe or cannula. Sometimes a cervical cap is used for a few hours to help keep the sperm from flowing out the vagina.

■ In IUI, the sperm are separated out of the seminal fluid. (This is necessary because seminal fluid contains chemicals that can irritate the uterus. Besides, separation selects the most motile sperm.) The sperm are then concentrated in a small volume of medium.

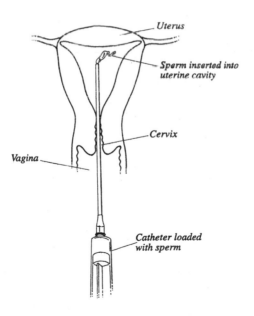

Uterus

Sperm inserted into
uterine cavity

Cervix

Vagina

Catheter loaded
with sperm

← Note!
Intrauterine
Insemination.
Washed sperm
are injected
through a
catheter into the
uterus.

Bright Idea
If you're plan-
ning on
therapeutic
insemination
using your part-
ner's sperm,
make sure he
tells the doctor
if he's had a
fever or
illness, which
can adversely
affect sperm
count, within the
last three
months. You'll
save yourself the
unnecessary test-
ing and drug
treatments that
are the conse-
quences of wast-
ing a cycle on
poor quality
sperm.

Rather than placing the washed sperm near the cervix, the sperm are loaded into a fine catheter that's inserted through the cervix into the uterus. The sperm are released high inside the uterus, even closer to the Fallopian tubes than possible with ICI. The procedure is usually painless. In recent years, IUI has replaced ICI as the technique of choice.

Another common problem for infertile couples is antisperm antibodies. Although more common in women, they can occur in men, as well. Several approaches to treating antisperm antibodies are available.

Other nonsurgical treatments of male infertility

As we saw in Chapter 2, male infertility can be caused by a number of conditions. It can't be overemphasized that the male partner must be as thoroughly evaluated as the female partner. A doctor specializing in male infertility (urologist or andrologist) should perform these evaluations. Any underlying medical condition, such as diabetes, must, of course, be treated.

Fertility drugs: not for women only

Although hormone deficiencies are relatively rare causes of male infertility, hormone replacement therapy is helping men with specific hormonal abnormalities. For example:

- Clomiphene citrate is used to stimulate sperm production.
- hMG (PERGONAL, HUMEGON, REPRONEX) are sometimes used to treat men with FSH and LH imbalances.
- hCG (PROFASI, PREGNYL, A.P.L.) is usually given along with hMG to stimulate the testicle to

produce testosterone and increase sperm production.

- Bromocriptine is used when it's certain that a man has hyperprolactinemia not caused by a pituitary tumor.

Antibiotics

Infection and inflammation of any of the glands or organs involved in sperm production and transport are not uncommon causes of male infertility. The prostate, seminal vesicles, epididymis, urethra, and even the testes themselves can be infected. Once an infection is diagnosed, and usually confirmed by a culture, an appropriately effective antibiotic is prescribed.

Other causes of male factor infertility

Retrograde ejaculation, in which semen is released backward into the bladder during ejaculation, can sometimes be overcome by either removing sperm from a urine sample and using it to inseminate the partner or by prescribing common over-the-counter oral medicines, such as the decongestant pseudoephedrine, which affects nerve signals and may help the bladder neck close during ejaculation, thus restoring antegrade, or normal, ejaculation.

If semen can't be deposited properly in the vagina because of a structural deformity of the penis, a problem called *hypospadias,* sometimes surgery can help correct the deformity. More often, however, TI is used.

For men suffering from neurologic defects or injuries that prevent them from ejaculating through sexual intercourse or masturbation, there are new *ejaculation stimulation* techniques to collect semen. Two primary ejaculatory stimulation methods are used:

Unofficially Heat may decrease sperm production in the testicles, so don't wear tight underwear or athletic supporters that hold the testicles too close to the body. Don't take hot baths or extended hot showers. Avoid long bike rides.

1. *Vibratory stimulation,* in which the penis is massaged with an electrically powered vibrating device.

2. *Electroejaculation stimulation (EES), in which* a probe is inserted into the rectum and a low level electrical current is supplied to excite the nerves and induce an ejaculation. (If the patient has rectal sensation, anesthesia is used.)

Just the facts

- Fertility drugs should never be taken for more than several months at a time.

- Fertility drugs should only be prescribed along with careful monitoring, including ultrasound and blood tests.

- Ideally, fertility drugs should not result in production of more than three or four eggs, unless you're planning to undergo an ART procedure.

GET THE SCOOP ON...
When surgery is appropriate ▪ Sterilization
reversals ▪ New sperm retrieval methods ▪
Factors to consider

Surgical Treatment for Infertility

Just a few years ago, surgery to correct many male and female infertility factors would have been out of the question or the outcome "iffy" at best for many couples. Reproductive organs may have been too damaged to repair with the then-available techniques, and surgeons did not have the tools that would allow them to work on such delicate tissues or in such confined areas.

But today's remarkable technical advances have overcome many of these obstacles. In fact, surgical techniques are now so refined that they are far less invasive, incapacitating, and painful than those performed just a few years ago. More importantly, most of them offer couples a real chance at restoring fertility. These advances include:

- Microsurgery, using high-power magnification, has made surgery on both the male and female reproductive organs feasible and successful.

- Lasers, which can remove diseased or damaged tissues with virtually no bleeding and trauma, have improved surgical outcomes.

- Endoscopic equipment, narrow fiberoptic instruments that allow doctors to look directly inside the body to examine damaged and diseased organs, have tremendous treatment applications, as well.

- Compact, precision instruments have been designed that allow surgeons to see, reach, and work within the confined spaces of the pelvis and other parts of the body.

- Micromanipulation techniques, which were developed for assisted reproductive technologies (ARTs) such as in vitro fertilization, have revolutionized the treatment of male factor infertility, in particular. (We'll be discussing these ART procedures in more detail in Chapter 7.)

Unofficially...
Although a woman may begin each cycle with several hundred eggs and follicles earmarked for development that month, the delicate hormonal balance only allows one or two to become fully developed and released. It's nature's way of assuring that humans have mainly single births.

The dilemma: to cut or not to cut

Ironically, these surgical advances have contributed to another sort of revolution in infertility management. Today, there's less reliance on surgery as a means of pursuing pregnancy than before.

Many couples, particularly older ones, now opt to skip conventional surgical procedures and go directly to high-tech ARTs to overcome infertility problems. Rather than trying to permanently restore fertility, they're choosing to temporarily bypass damaged and poorly functioning reproductive organs to achieve conception. These procedures are giving older couples, as well as couples in which the woman has had extensive tubal damage, a better chance at conceiving and having a healthy baby than traditional surgeries do.

Nevertheless, before going to the ARTs, many couples are still helped by the conventional surgeries we'll talk about in this chapter. You and your partner may have a problem that is quite amenable to surgical correction. So it's important to explore all your options with your doctor.

Surgery is less invasive than ever before

The good news about today's surgical procedures to correct infertility is that they're often less invasive and traumatic than ever before. This translates into less pain and discomfort, faster recuperation, and often, better results.

This is clearly evident in the case of some of the newer technologies. For example, one exciting advance in infertility treatment has been the expanded use of *endoscopic* equipment, which was designed originally for diagnosis but is now being used during surgery. Doctors now can not only inspect your internal organs up-close, but they can correct many problems they see as soon as they're found, obviating the need for a second or more invasive procedure, referred to as open surgery.

The two endoscopic instruments used commonly in minimally invasive infertility surgery are laparoscopes and hysteroscopes, which you may remember from the discussion in Chapter 4 on diagnosis. When these pieces of fiberoptic equipment are used to diagnose or evaluate a problem, the procedures are called *diagnostic laparoscopy* or *diagnostic hysteroscopy*. When used to fix a problem, they're called *operative laparoscopy* or *operative hysteroscopy*. Operative laparoscopies have largely replaced open, abdominal surgeries for many types of infertility problems, particularly tubal repair. Hysteroscopic surgery eliminates the need to cut through major organs. These instruments are being used to correct many uterine disorders, including uterine endometriosis and fibroids.

You've already read about these two techniques in their diagnostic mode; here's how they're used operatively:

- Laparoscopes are inserted through a small incision at or near your "belly button." Your doctor will inspect your uterus, Fallopian tubes, and ovaries. If a correctable problem is discovered, operative instruments, such as laser equipment, surgical knives, and sutures, can be inserted through other small abdominal incisions.

- Hysteroscopes allow doctors to view your uterus and Fallopian tubes from the inside through a thin, telescopic instrument passed through the vagina and cervix. Again, if a correctable problem is uncovered, operative instruments can be passed through the hysteroscope. For example, if a minor blockage is seen, a flexible tube or wire is slid through the hysteroscope and used to push or scrape out the blockage. Hysteroscopic surgery can also be used to remove some types of fibroids and septum defects.

These procedures are usually done with you as an outpatient. You won't be incapacitated but will probably be told to rest for the next few days or week. You won't need much more than mild analgesics and antibiotics.

On the other hand, traditional surgeries require general anesthesia and are highly invasive. The surgeon must make a fairly large incision in your abdomen just to reach organs needing repair. These newer procedures are far less invasive. While sometimes these endoscopic approaches take time,

Watch Out!
If you've had tubal disease, you must see your doctor as soon as you think you may be pregnant. Even if you've had tubal repair done, your chances of have an ectopic pregnancy are higher than normal. You need to undergo tests to determine exactly where the embryo is.

you're organs are far less traumatized. You need less—and less powerful—medication.

Surgical solutions

Whether open or minimally invasive, surgery still has an important place in the treatment of female-factor infertility, including tubal, pelvic or uterine, and ovarian infertility.

Tubal disease or obstructions

Tubal disease is one of the most common causes of female infertility, accounting for one quarter to one-third of cases. Tubal disease usually means tubal obstructions, and unblocking these obstructions is one of the most common indications for surgery. As we discussed in Chapter 2, the causes of tubal disease vary and include:

- **Scarring and adhesions.** These are usually due to infections or previous surgeries. A common and growing cause are sexually transmitted diseases (STDs), as we saw in Chapter 4. In addition, STDs increase your risk of pelvic inflammatory disease (PID), which can be devastating to the entire female reproductive tract. Tubal adhesions sometimes result from endometriosis.

- **Endometriosis.** Misplaced endometrial tissue can lodge and grow in and around the Fallopian tubes and cause tubal obstructions. Endometrial tissue can also end up at other sites in the abdominal cavity, particularly the uterus. Scar tissue can build up, bind, and block reproductive structures needed for conception and pregnancy. (See the discussion of surgery for pelvic endometriosis and adhesions later in this chapter.)

Moneysaver
Talk to your doctor *and* insurance company before undergoing an exploratory laparoscopy. If your doctor ends up recommending an ART, but your insurance doesn't cover it but does cover laparoscopic tubal repair, that may be your only financial option. You'll want to know before going into the test so that the repair can be done at the same time as the exploratory laparoscopy.

■ **Tubal ligation or sterilization.** This is a common form of contraception designed to permanently block an egg from traveling down and sperm from swimming up the Fallopian tubes.

As you learned in Chapter 4, sometimes a diagnostic procedure done to *evaluate* tubal blockage can actually result in its repair. This is particularly true if the blockages are minor and located proximally—that is, if the blockage is found in the part of the Fallopian tube that is nearest to the uterus. (Distal blockages are closer to the ends of the Fallopian tubes—that is, they occur near the ovaries.) In addition, a repair can be performed during certain types of diagnostic procedures, like exploratory laparoscopy.

One diagnostic procedure, an X-ray called the *hysterosalpingogram,* has been known to correct some tubal obstructions in one of two ways:

■ During the procedure, a radio-opaque dye is injected through the cervix into the uterus and Fallopian tubes. Just the pressure of the dye traveling through the tubes can sometimes open tiny blockages.

■ The radiologist who performs the hysterosalpingogram will snake very thin catheters up the uterus into your Fallopian tubes in a procedure called *transcervical cannulation,* or *tubal catheterization.* By flushing fluid or passing a wire through the catheters, a proximal blockage may be opened.

In addition, a hysteroscopy or laparoscopy can be used as a means to gain access into the reproductive structures and undertake repairs.

When more is needed

Unfortunately, not all tubal repairs can be done through these minimally invasive approaches. For more extensive tubal repairs, like the tubal sterilization reversal we discussed earlier, laparotomies are required.

The location of your obstruction dictates the particular type of laparotomy surgery you'll need. Here are three of the most common surgical options:

- **Salpingostomy** is a procedure in which a cut is made in the fimbrial end of the Fallopian tube and blockages or damaged tissues are removed.

- **Fimbrostomy** is a procedure that corrects any damage to the actual fimbria.

- **Tubal reimplantation** removes the Fallopian tube from the uterus and reconnects it to the uterine wall.

Reversing tubal sterilization

Tubal obstructions are not the only reasons women need tubal surgery. About 10 percent of all women who've undergone *tubal sterilization*, sometimes called *tubal ligation* or "having your tubes tied," later change their minds. Reversing female sterilization, commonly known as "untying the tubes," is usually successful—that is, it opens the tubes—in about 75 to 90 percent of the cases. But pregnancy rates are lower—only between 60 to 75 percent of women who have their tubal ligations reversed succeed in getting pregnant. Three factors help to determine success in reversing the sterilization:

- How the original tubal ligation was done. If rings or clips were used to block off the Fallopian tubes, you've probably had less tubal

Timesaver
Before undergoing a specialized diagnostic test, like an exploratory laparoscopy or hysteroscopy, ask if the person doing the test can also make repairs right then and there. You don't always have to reschedule a corrective procedure after the diagnostic test.

damage than if the sterilization was done by actually destroying your tubes with *electrocautery.* If your tubes were tied in their midsection, you can expect a good outcome.

■ How much of the tubes remain after the reversal. The more Fallopian tube left, the better the chances for pregnancy.

■ How experienced the surgeon is. The reversal of a tubal sterilization is an exacting surgery using microsurgical techniques. You need to find a qualified surgeon who specializes in this type of microsurgery. The more experience the surgeon has had in doing this surgery, the more likely the success.

Tubal ligation reversal involves a *laparotomy,* which is a major open surgical procedure. You'll need general anesthesia. In the laparotomy, the surgeon cuts through the abdomen to get to the Fallopian tubes. Working with microsurgical instruments, the surgeon then cuts out the damaged portion of the tubes and sews the remaining sections back together again.

You'll probably be in the hospital for a few days after the laparotomy, and painkillers will most likely be in order. After discharge, you'll probably be laid up for several weeks recuperating.

Obviously, this is significant surgery. It is therefore important that you talk to your doctor about the relative risks and benefits of having this procedure done. There are alternatives—particularly in the field of assisted reproductive technology (ART). Table 6.1 gives a quick comparison of surgery and ART for tubal disease.

**TABLE 6.1: A COMPARISON OF SURGERY
TO ARTs AS TREATMENT FOR TUBAL DISEASE:
THE PROS AND CONS**

	Surgery	ART
Invasive	More	Less
Cost	Less	More
Recuperation	Lengthy	Minimal
Success	Somewhat better	Not as good
Future success	Allows continued attempts at pregnancy	Permits attempts only through treatment cycles
Insurance coverage	Usually	Questionable
Fertility drugs	No	Yes

Endometriosis and other pelvic adhesions

Pelvic endometriosis and pelvic adhesions (scar tissue) are other common causes of female infertility. And, like several other female infertility factors for which extensive surgery was standard, their current surgical management includes less invasive measures than were required in the past.

Endometriosis is the build-up of little implants of tissue outside the uterus. When the tissue lodges in the ovary it can cause ovarian cysts, called *endometriomas*. In addition, endometriosis can lead to tubal or pelvic adhesions as endometrial tissue irritates surrounding structures. (Adhesions can also result from infections, injuries, or previous abdominal surgery.) Although frequently treated with hormonal drugs, such as danazol or gonadotropin-releasing hormone agonists (such as GnRH-a), endometriosis is sometimes severe enough to require surgery, or surgery plus drug therapy. If the doctor finds endometriosis during diagnostic laparoscopy, which is the only definitive way to tell if, indeed, you do have it, the endometriosis tissue can be vaporized, using lasers or electric current. (See Chapter 5 for more information about the medical treatment of endometriosis.)

In the past, laparotomy, a form of open abdominal surgery, was used extensively to help reduce pelvic adhesions. But success using this technique was limited, because the open abdominal surgery itself could lead to scarring, and cutting out or scraping away the adhesions would itself cause new, albeit sometimes smaller, scars to form. Today, the laparoscopic removal of pelvic adhesions—usually using a laser and/or electric current—is the treatment of choice. This less invasive technique only requires small incisions, and the lasers and/or electric current used to vaporize the adhesions makes cutting them out unnecessary.

Today, when laparotomy is needed to remove scar tissue, there are ways surgeons have found to help reduce recurrence, too. These include taking medications, such as anti-inflammatory drugs and antibiotics. Some surgeons advocate irrigating the pelvic cavity with a sterile solution during surgery and filling it before they close you up. This ensures that no small blood clots are left behind to start a new inflammatory reaction, and it allows your organs to float freely without bumping into each other for a day or two immediately following the operation. Absorbable materials can also be used to cover the internal surgical site to help prevent adhesion formation.

Removing uterine fibroids

Uterine fibroids, sometimes called *uterine myomas*, are one of the more common uterine disorders contributing to infertility, affecting about 20 to 25 percent of American women. These abnormal, but noncancerous, masses of smooth muscle tissue can prevent an embryo from implanting or growing in the womb. Location is everything when it comes to uterine fibroids. *Submucosal* fibroids grow inside the uterine cavity and pose the biggest threat to pregnancy.

Uterine fibroids can be removed during an operative (as opposed to diagnostic) hysteroscopy, an operative laparoscopy, or on occasion by laparotomy. But be aware that you shouldn't need to have your uterus removed to treat these growths. A hysterectomy is decidedly *not* the first treatment option to consider.

Surgical correction of male factor infertility

While the ARTs have replaced many surgeries to correct female factor infertility, surgery for male factor infertility is actually increasing. In fact, some of the new sperm retrieval procedures to help overcome male factor infertility have their roots in the micromanipulation techniques that were refined for use in the ARTs.

Vasectomy reversal

Vasectomy has long been a safe, effective, popular—and once nonreversible—contraceptive method for men in this country. But, as with female sterilization, many men are also seeking to reverse their sterility. Over the last two decades, *vasectomy reversal*, sometimes called a *microsurgical repair of vasal obstruction*, has been refined—and success rates are getting better.

One key consideration affecting the chances of successful reversal is the length of time since the

Moneysaver
Because vasectomy reversals are much less expensive than sperm retrieval and ICSI procedures, you might choose an attempt at vasectomy reversal before opting to go on to the high-tech procedures, particularly if you have the time to wait for a pregnancy.

vasectomy was done. The best results—obviously measured in terms of the ability to produce a pregnancy—are achieved if the sterilization was performed within the last ten years. But it's not unheard of for vasectomies performed twenty years ago to be reversed successfully. And if the vasectomy was done less than three years ago, you could be looking at a pregnancy rate of about 75 percent.

Depending or your particular situation there are two microsurgical procedures that can be performed for vasectomy reversal: *vasovasotomy* and *vasoepididymostomy* which we'll discuss in greater detail later.

Correcting Obstructive Azoospermia

You might also undergo these procedures if you have what's called obstructive azoospermia, a condition in which no sperm are found in the ejaculate because of some type of blockage. The blockage might be something present from birth or gotten due to any number of reasons, like a hernia. If that's the case, you'll under go a few more tests before having one of the microsurgical procedures mentioned earlier. Careful reading of the test results can help pinpoint the exact location of a blockage. Besides a physical exam and semen analysis, your FSH blood and seminal fluctose levels should be tested, as well. You'll probably have a testicular biopsy taken to show if indeed you're producing sperm. The FSH tests are very important: If your FSH levels are very high, you're probably not producing any sperm. An attempt at reversal would therefore be pointless.

If your semen has fructose in it, on the other hand, your seminal vesicles are most likely working normally. If your testes are producing sperm but there are no sperm in the semen, the obstruction is no doubt located somewhere between the testes and the urethra.

Vasovasotomy is the most common vasectomy-reversal surgery currently being performed and it's simpler to do—and say—than a vasoepididymostomy. It's goal is to remove the sections of the vas deferens that were destroyed during the original sterilization procedure and are now blocking sperm transport and to reconnect the clean open ends. (For a reminder of the physical details of the male reproductive system, refer to Chapter 1.)

In this exacting surgery, small incisions are made in each side of the scrotum. Depending on exactly where along the vas the original vasectomy was done, the incision may have to be extended higher, and the surgeon might need to bring the testes and epididymis out of the scrotum to work on them.

The damaged vas deferens portions are cut out. Before reconnecting the two clean ends, your surgeon will make a few critical observations and determinations. First, your doctor will want to verify that sperm are present. To do this some fluid is removed from the vas deferens and examined under a microscope. If sperm or parts of sperm are found in the fluid, the operation can proceed normally. This involves stitching back together both the inner and outer layers of the tube-like vas. The idea is that sperm will once again travel freely through the vas deferens and out the urethra during ejaculation.

But it may be the case that no sperm are found in the vas fluid. If no sperm are present, your surgeon will probably opt to perform a vasoepididymostomy—a more complicated procedure. This happens in about one-third of vasovasotomy cases.

Unofficially... Annually, about a half million American men undergo vasectomies. An estimated one percent of them will change their minds each year—and the percent is rising. The reasons are plentiful: a new marriage, death of a child, or just wanting more children.

Vasoepididymostomy is performed if an obstruction has formed in the epididymal tubule. An obstruction sometimes develops if testicular fluid builds up after a vasectomy. It can also occur after an infection or injury. Sometimes it's due to a congenital defect.

Vasoepididymostomy is designed to bypass the obstructed area in the epididymal tubules. Instead of sewing the two ends of the vas back together after the removal of the damaged portion, one end is stitched directly to the epididymal tubules, above the point of the obstruction. The other end of the vas is left behind. This allows sperm to flow from the epididymis directly into the vas deferens, bypassing the blockage.

What to expect

Both of these surgeries, which can last for a couple of hours, are done as outpatient procedures with local or general anesthesia. You may be told to stay in bed for a day or so and not to resume strenuous physical or sexual activity for two to six weeks. You'll be given mild analgesics and maybe an antibiotic. After about six to eight weeks, you'll undergo monthly semen analyses to check on results.

Your doctor may be able to get some idea during surgery about how successful the procedures will be. Pregnancy rates following vasectomy seem to correlate with the quality of the sperm seen in the vas deferens fluid during surgery. The more motile sperm, the better the likely outcome.

Most pregnancies occur within two years after a successful vasectomy reversal. If your semen analysis after the reversal is good but no pregnancy has occurred, you should be tested for antisperm antibodies. Nearly three-quarters of men who have had a vasectomy develop antisperm antibodies. But because vasectomy reversals tend to turn out so well, antisperm antibody testing isn't routinely done. It's really a poor predictor of whether pregnancy can be achieved after surgery.

And, of course, your partner needs to continue to be evaluated. She may have developed a fertility-related problem in the meantime.

Fixing a varicocele

Varicoceles, or varicose veins surronding the testicles, are quite common, particularly in men who suffer from infertility. About 10 to 15 percent of all men have varicoceles, but the rate is much higher for men who are infertile: about 30 to 40 percent of men who go to the doctor for an infertility evaluation have this condition.

What to expect

Varicocelectomy is a relatively simple and commonly performed surgery to correct this cause of male factor infertility. It is performed as an outpatient procedure with local, regional, or general anesthesia. The surgeon makes a small incision in the groin and ties off the enlarged veins.

Semen quality seems to improve in some men undergoing this procedure. Unfortunately, it's hard to predict who'll be helped and who won't. A review of nearly 3,000 cases in one of the largest male infertility centers in the country showed that semen quality improved in about two-thirds of the men having surgery, and about 40 percent successfully impregnated their partners.

Opening blocked ejaculatory ducts

A procedure called *transurethral resection of the ejaculatory duct (TURED)*, is performed to open a

Bright Idea
If you're planning a vasectomy reversal, ask your doctor if sperm can be removed and frozen for later use. If the reversal doesn't work, at least you may get enough sperm to produce a pregnancy later.

blockage, which may be the result of infection or a congenital abnormality, in the complex systems of ducts leading from the testes to the urethra. Depending on where along the sperm transport route the blockage is, either microsurgery or endoscopic surgical repair is possible. TURED is usually highly successful in correcting this type of male infertility problem. The procedure takes only about 30 minutes and it's done with an instrument that passes through the urethra in the penis.

New sperm retrieval techniques

Today, men who have too few sperm (*oligospermia*) or no sperm at all (*azoospermia*) in their ejaculate—including those who have had unsuccessful vasectomy reversals—are being helped through highly advanced microsurgical techniques. These procedures allow for direct sperm retrieval from men who, just a few years ago, had virtually no chance of fathering a child. Keep in mind that there are two types of azoospermia:

1. *Obstructive azoospermia.* In this condition, the testes produce sperm but their transport is somehow blocked.

2. *Nonobstructive azoospermia.* In this case, it's not blockage that's the problem. It's that the testes are producing too few, if any, sperm.

Recently, several techniques have been developed to help men with obstructive and nonobstructive azoospermia. These procedures are used in combination with a technique called *intracytoplasmic sperm injection (ICSI)*, either performed immediately or at a later time with frozen sperm. (See Chapter 7 for more information about ICSI.) The

Bright Idea
If you're going to undergo one of the new sperm retrieval methods, talk to your doctor about whether sperm can be frozen for later use. This would allow another attempt when the woman has a good quality ovulation.

new procedures include:

- *Microsurgical epididymal sperm aspiration (MESA).* This microsurgical technique is used to retrieve sperm in men with obstructive azoospermia. This occurs in men who have been born without the vas deferens or who have blocked vas deferens. Sperm are removed directly from the epididymis.

  In this procedure, an incision is made in the scrotum and—using micropipettes or cannulas—either a small incision or a puncture is made into the individual tubules of the epididymis. If moving sperm are found in the tubule, the fluid is collected and used immediately for ICSI. (You can have some sperm frozen for later use, as well.)

  This technique is particularly helpful for men who have had a vasectomy that cannot be reversed or certain congenital abnormalities, or who suffer from a neurologic disorder or injury that prevents ejaculation.

- *Percutaneous epididymal sperm aspiration (PESA)* is a simpler, less invasive procedure than MESA and is also used to retrieve sperm from men with obstructive azoospermia. In PESA a needle is used to repeatedly puncture the epididymis to aspirate sperm. Sperm collected this way are also used immediately in an ICSI procedure.

- *Testicular sperm extraction (TESE)* is helping men with obstructive or nonobstructive azoospermia. In this procedure, sperm are extracted using a biopsy needle directly from the testicular tissue through a small incision made in the scrotum. A piece of testicular tissue is

Watch Out!
If you have nonobstructive azoospermia but don't know what's the cause, talk to your doctor about genetic screening to help identify any genetic abnormalities that might be responsible for the condition. If you have obstructed azoospermia and were born without vas deferens, you should be tested for cystic fibrosis gene mutations.

removed and examined in the lab to see if sperm are there. If they are, the sperm can be used immediately in an ICSI procedure or frozen for later use.

■ *Percutaneous testicular sperm aspiration (TESA)* involves puncturing the testes repeatedly with a needle, aspirating the sperm, and using them immediately in an ICSI procedure. This procedure is usually reserved for men with obstructive azoospermia since so few sperm are available in nonobstructive azoospermia that only actually removing testicular tissue in TESE will yield enough sperm for an ICSI procedure.

Making the decision to have surgery

As you can see, you often have several options in the surgical treatment of male and female infertility. Some involve deciding between traditional and minimally invasive surgeries. Others involve choosing between any surgery at all and an assisted reproductive technology.

So, before undergoing any surgical correction of an infertility problem you need to have a frank discussion with your infertility specialist and/or your surgeon. You should examine the pros and cons of any procedure and discuss all the options that are available, both at your infertility center and at others.

It's important to remember that all of these microsurgical procedures require surgical expertise. So if you need to undergo microsurgery for your infertility, it's important that you find a surgeon with a good track record for the specific procedure you need. Ask, "How often do you do this procedure?" "What's your success rate with this type of procedure?" "What's the success rate nationally or at other centers?"

In particular, a highly experienced surgeon is needed because, for many types of surgeries, and particularly for tubal repairs, one attempt at correction is usually all that can and should be tried. Repeated microsurgical corrections are not very successful.

With any surgery, there are certain questions that you're well-advised to ask, such as: "How long will the surgery take?" and "How long will I be in the hospital?" If the surgery is done with you as an outpatient, find out how long you're actually going to be at the facility so you can make appropriate arrangements for transportation.

There are other important questions to ask to make your recovery easier. Here's a helpful list to take with you when you're discussing a surgical option with your doctor:

- How much pain should I expect?

- What painkillers can I take? (Of course, get a prescription for any painkillers or antibiotics you might need *before* you leave the facility at which your surgery is done. In fact, some facilities have on-site pharmacies that will fill a small prescription to tide you over until you can get a full prescription filled.)

- What kind of follow-up care will I need?

- How long will I be laid up?

- When can I resume nonstrenuous activities? Strenuous ones?

- When can I go back to work?

Finally, ask what follow-up tests, if any, you might need. And, of course, find out when you can expect to see results from the surgery.

While you're having your preliminary discussions about surgery with your regular physician, remember that it's always a good idea to get a second opinion before undergoing infertility surgery. Reputable surgeons won't mind, and insurance carriers usually require it.

Just the facts

- Today's remarkable technological advances have made it possible to correct many formerly untreatable forms of infertility.

- Surgical procedures to correct infertility are far less invasive and traumatic than ever before.

- In some cases, diagnostic procedures can themselves serve to reverse some conditions of infertility.

- Tubal ligations and vasectomies are now being reversed surgically with encouragingly high rates of success.

- Modern sperm retrieval techniques are making it possible for many men to successfully father a biological child who would not have been able to just a few short years ago.

Assisted Reproductive Technologies

GET THE SCOOP ON...
What's new in the ARTs ▪ Who should
consider the ARTs ▪ From IVF to ZIFT ▪
New frontiers in the ARTs

PART IV

Chapter 7

The State of the ARTs

It's been two decades since the world's first so-called "test-tube" baby, Louise Brown, was born in England. Assisted reproductive technology (ART) has come a long way since then!

Louise Brown was conceived through *in vitro fertilization (IVF)*, a technique in which eggs and sperm are mixed (in a Petri dish, not a test-tube!) If fertilization takes place and the fertilized egg begins dividing, the resulting embryo is transferred to the mother's uterus, where, hopefully, it will implant and result in pregnancy.

Since that first successful and classic IVF procedure, the ARTs have been refined and spin-off procedures have been developed that are helping tens of thousands of infertile couples, who would have had little or no hope of having their own biological child, realize their dream.

Who are the ARTs helping?

Initially, IVF was developed, and for some time viewed, as a last resort to help women who had blocked, injured, or no Fallopian tubes to conceive.

Unofficially...
More than 92,000 babies— 59,000 of whom were conceived through IVF, the first ART used in this country— have been born in the United States as a result of ARTs. Despite these numbers, less than 5 percent of all infertile couples who enter infertility treatment will undergo these advanced procedures.

While ARTs are still being used largely to treat tubal factor infertility, their uses are expanding. And they are being used earlier in the treatment of infertility.

Couples with unexplained infertility, men with low or no sperm counts, and older women are among the groups now realizing success through ARTs. Table 7.1 shows the primary indications for ART procedures performed in 1996 and how successful ARTs were based on these diagnoses. Keep in mind that these were primary diagnoses only and that couples probably had more than one factor contributing to their infertility Also, these data are from 1995. Most fertility experts agree that success rates are considerably higher now.

TABLE 7.1: PRIMARY DIAGNOSES AND LIVE BIRTH RATES IN COUPLES USING THEIR OWN FRESH SPERM AND EGGS IN ART PROCEDURES (1996)

Cause	Percent of Patients	Success Rate
Tubal factor	29%	21.6%
Male factor	25%	24.3%
Endometriosis	16%	23.8%
Unexplained	8%	23.0%
Ovarian factor	12%	21.8%
Uterine	2%	17.0%
Other	8%	20.1%

Source: *American Society for Reproductive Medicine, 1996.*

In general, you and your doctor will take into account three main medical issues when considering whether the ARTs are appropriate for you:

- **Your age.** By now you know that conception is harder and almost any infertility treatment is less likely to be successful the older you are. So if you're older you may not have the luxury of time to try more conventional treatments.

- The length of time you've been trying to conceive with conventional treatments. Maybe it's time to consider other approaches.

- Your chances of success with both less expensive or less invasive procedures and with ARTs.

We'll be looking later at what else to consider before deciding on an ART procedure, and, we'll give you some tips on how to choose an ART program. Before we do that, it will help for you to know what's involved in ART procedures. We'll give you a handle on the subtle differences between the procedures that have evolved from the original IVF technology, and the newly developed sperm and egg micromanipulation techniques.

Knowing the scope of the options available will make you better prepared to choose an ART program that's right for you. Some ARTs are best suited for specific female or male factor infertilities. Some work well when both partners have problems, and it's not usual to find that after one ART method fails, another is tried. Keep in mind when looking for an ART program that what you think you need today may not be what you know you'll need tomorrow.

What you can expect

There are several key steps to IVF and its closely related offspring—GIFT (gamete intrafallopian transfer), ZIFT (zygote intrafallopian transfer), and TET (tubal embryo transfer). The latest micromanipulation techniques are really adjuncts to these procedures, so the overall steps in all these treatments are the same. They are:

1. Ovulation induction

2. Egg retrieval

Timesaver
Besides this *Unofficial Guide*, collect materials about ART programs from specialty medical societies and patient advocate groups, such as RESOLVE. Call for information packets from programs in your area and around the country. You'll learn more about all the choices, which will save time in finding programs that will meet your needs today and tomorrow.

66

In high school, when kids would call Louise Brown a test-tube baby, she was quick to retort: 'I'm a test-tube teenager!'

99

3. Fertilization

4. Embryo transfer

5. Implantation

Ovulation induction is used to stimulate the ovaries to produce several mature eggs in one cycle. The chance for pregnancy is greater if more than one egg is available for fertilization and transfer to the woman's uterus. (See Chapter 5 for more information about the role of fertility drugs in the treatment of infertility.)

As we saw in Chapter 5, a critical component in ovulation induction is timing. Therefore, you must go to a program that has 24-hour-a-day, 365-day-a-year, availability. (There will be more later on what to look for in an ART program.)

You'll be returning to the facility several times for blood tests and ultrasound monitoring to pinpoint when follicles are maturing and to watch for ovarian hyperstimulation syndrome.

Note! ➔
Egg retrieval with an ultra-sound-guided needle. In egg retrieval, ripe eggs from the follicles of an ovary are aspirated through a needle that is inserted through the vagina, guided by an ultrasound probe.

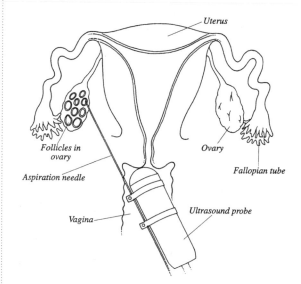

Uterus

Follicles in ovary

Ovary

Aspiration needle

Fallopian tube

Vagina

Ultrasound probe

Then you'll be given other hormones to induce follicle release and an egg retrieval session will be scheduled. If all goes according to plan, eggs are retrieved and an embryo transfer is performed. You may also be given progesterone to help make the uterine environment more receptive to implantation.

As we saw in Chapter 5, successful ovulation induction is tantamount to a hormonal balancing act and is as much an art as a science. That's one reason why not all ovulation induction cycles end in retrievals and, therefore, not all end in fertilization and embryo transfers. Despite the common use of GnRH agonists, which help prevent premature ovulation and inadvertent loss of follicles before retrieval, about 15 percent of cycles are cancelled before retrieval and more than 23 percent before transfer.

Occasionally an approach called *natural cycle IVF,* in which no fertility drugs are given, is used. It has several advantages as well as drawbacks. It's cheaper and requires less monitoring than ovulation induction, and of course, it carries none of risks of fertility drugs, like ovarian hyperstimulation. On the other hand, you need to know that you ovulate and only one egg is available for retrieval at a time. Success rates per cycle are much lower than for ovulation-induced IVF procedures.

The what's, when's, where's, and how's of IVF procedures

GIFT, ZIFT, and TET are variations of the classic IVF procedure. They differ in the way eggs are retrieved, where fertilization takes place, what is transferred, and where it goes.

For example, IVF waits until a fertilized egg has divided several times before transfer into the uterus; GIFT doesn't wait for fertilization to occur before transferring the eggs and sperm into the Fallopian tubes. IVF relies on transvaginal retrieval and transfer while GIFT uses a laparoscopic approach.

These and other differences allow your doctor to choose the treatment that's best for you. Some factors that you and your doctor will consider when choosing one of the IVF procedures are the status of your Fallopian tubes, whether you know your eggs can be fertilized, whether you have mild or severe endometriosis, and whether you produce sperm antibodies and, if so, how severe the condition is.

For example, if your Fallopian tubes are blocked, GIFT is not for you. Nor may GIFT be right for you if your partner's sperm quality is poor. But if you have mild endometriosis or unexplained infertility, GIFT may be a good choice. Today, because IVF does not require surgery and its pregnancy rate is equal to or higher than GIFT, ZIFT, or TET, IVF is done almost exclusively.

Defining the ARTs

Now that you know the key steps in the IVF procedures as well as their overall differences, it's time to take a more detailed look at each technique.

In vitro fertilization (IVF)

In this classic ART, a woman is given fertility drugs to produce several eggs, which are retrieved from the ovaries in one of two ways—by transvaginal ultrasound aspiration or occasionally, laparoscopy.

In *transvaginal ultrasound aspiration*, which is usually performed with local anesthesia or under mild sedation, an ultrasound probe inserted through the vagina sends back high-frequency

Unofficially...
It's progesterone that causes the temperature rise following ovulation, and it's progesterone that sustains a pregnancy. Maybe Mother Nature was trying to create a nice, warm place for a fetus to grow!

sound waves to identify mature follicles. If such follicles are found, a special narrow needle is guided through the vagina to the ovaries to suck up, or aspirate, the follicles. During *laparoscopic aspiration*, which is performed under general anesthesia, the doctor inserts a narrow, telescopic device through a small incision in or below the woman's navel. If mature eggs are seen, the doctor guides a needle through the abdominal wall to retrieve them.

Regardless of the aspiration technique employed, each retrieved egg is mixed with the man's sperm, which have been separated from their seminal fluid through a process called *sperm washing*. The mixing is done in a lab dish containing a special culture medium. The mixture is then placed in an incubator set to the same temperature as a woman's body. If fertilization occurs and the cultured embryo starts dividing, a transfer is scheduled, usually in three to four days when the embryo reaches about an eight-cell stage or beyond.

Embryo transfer is done as an outpatient procedure without anesthesia (although sometimes the woman is given a mild sedative). The embryos and some of the culture media are loaded into a special catheter, which is inserted through the cervix into the uterus. There they are gently deposited and, it is hoped, one successfully implants itself on the uterine wall.

To increase the chances of success, more than one embryo is transferred at a time—most commonly two or three. Extra embryos can be cryopreserved for transfer during another cycle if pregnancy doesn't occur after the initial transfer.

Pregnancy rates vary from center to center, and by underlying condition. Older women, those with poor uterine environments, and those whose

Bright Idea
The American Society of Reproductive Medicine recommends that you and your doctor agree on how many embryos to transfer and you sign an informed consent. Because of financial considerations, some couples choose to have more than a few embryos transferred, but this raises the risk of multiple gestations. When faced with this situation, some couples opt for selective reduction. But, this is an issue that you, your partner, and your doctor must discuss in advance.

partners have poor sperm quality are less likely to have success.

Gamete intrafallopian transfer (GIFT)

In gamete intrafallopian transfer, eggs can be retrieved as in IVF by transvaginal aspiration, or laparoscopically. Then the retrieved eggs and sperm are mixed together. In GIFT, however, they're placed directly into one or both Fallopian tubes, rather than off in a petri dish full of culture medium. It's hoped that fertilization will occur while the mixed sperm and eggs are in the tubes. (Sometimes doctors wait a few minutes to give sperm time to attach to an egg's outer shell before transferring the mixture.)

Some couples find GIFT a more natural, and therefore more philosophically appealing, method for conception, since fertilization takes place within the woman's body. In the past, GIFT worked better than IVF for some couples. But since pregnancy rates with IVF have steadily increased over the years (in most programs they equal or are better than GIFT), GIFT is being used less and less often. Another consideration is that GIFT, as well as ZIFT, which we will discuss next, require laparoscopy. IVF does not.

GIFT is only an option for women with normal Fallopian tubes. Women with mild endometriosis are also candidates for GIFT. Because it's impossible to determine fertilization—unless a pregnancy occurs—GIFT is not used unless it's known that the sperm can fertilize an egg.

Zygote intrafallopian transfer (ZIFT)

ZIFT is sometimes known as *PROST (pronuclear stage transfer)* and can best be understood as an IVF-GIFT hybrid. It's not widely used, if at all, today. As in IVF, eggs are retrieved transvaginally and mixed with sperm in the lab. If fertilization occurs, resulting zygotes, which are fertilized but undivided eggs, are transferred via laparoscopy, as in GIFT, into the Fallopian tubes within about twenty-four hours. As we said earlier with GIFT, IVF success is obviating the need to use ZIFT and it eliminates the need for a laparoscopy.

If the quality of the woman's eggs is in doubt, ZIFT is sometimes advised over GIFT because fertilization can be detected. If GIFT fails, ZIFT might be tried.

Tubal embryo transfer (TET)

This is another IVF-GIFT combination technique. Like ZIFT, it's not widely used today. As in IVF, more developed (four-to-eight cell stage) fertilized eggs are transferred. But, as in GIFT, embryos are transferred into the Fallopian tubes.

Micromanipulation techniques

Micromanipulation techniques are allowing doctors to work with individual embryos and sperm.

- *Assisted hatching.* In this micromanipulation technique, an acidic solution is used to delicately open an embryo's outer cover, or zona pellucida. The embryo is then washed, replaced in the culture medium, and incubated. Shortly thereafter, the embryo is transferred.

  Assisted hatching may help a normal, growing embryo emerge from its natural covering and implant itself more easily in the uterus. But it's also being used when cell division is slow, and on embryos with thick outer shells. It seems to help improve the chance of implantation, particularly in older women.

Moneysaver
If you're planning a GIFT procedure, talk to your doctor about mixing any extra eggs with sperm in the lab (as in a standard IVF procedure). Cryopreserve embryos that develop. If you don't get pregnant from the GIFT procedure, you can elect later to thaw the embryos and do a transfer. You won't need another round of ovulation induction or egg retrieval. This can save you both money and time.

▪ *Intracytoplasmic sperm injection (ICSI)*. Although pioneered only in the early 1990s, ICSI is now one of the most successful of the micromanipulation methods and is being performed by most IVF centers in this country. (ICSI has replaced earlier techniques, such as partial zona dissection [PZD] and subzonal sperm insemination [SUSI], which sought to get sperm past an egg's hard outer surface.)

In this procedure, the woman undergoes ovulation induction and egg retrieval. The man provides a semen specimen (either through masturbation, ejaculatory stimulation, or sperm aspiration.) From this specimen, one sperm is drawn into a microscopic needle and injected directly into a single egg. This is done until all the mature eggs are injected or all the functional sperm are used up. If fertilization occurs, resulting embryos are transferred, as in an IVF procedure, into the woman's uterus.

Before the ARTs, the only options available for men with low sperm counts were artificial insemination, adoption, or child-free living. In the last few years, micromanipulation and sperm aspiration techniques have made it possible, however, for men with very low sperm counts or those unable to provide semen specimens to father children. (See Chapter 5 for more information on ejaculatory stimulation and Chapter 6 for more information on sperm aspiration.)

Unlike previous approaches to male factor infertility that focused on increasing the quantity or quality of sperm, micromanipulation focuses on an individual sperm. In essence, as long as there is one good, viable sperm, which is all that nature needs or allows anyway, fertilization can occur.

ICSI is being used to help men who were born without the vas deferens, the conduit that transports sperm from the testis, or men who have obstructions that can't be repaired, and those with severely decreased sperm counts to father children. It has greatly reduced the use of, therapeutic, or artificial insemination with donor sperm.

Cryopreservation: an expanding frontier in ART

Human sperm have been frozen successfully and used for more than forty years. Human embryos have been successfully cryopreserved, thawed, and implanted for the last fifteen years. But, human eggs have been a completely different story—until very recently.

▪ *Frozen sperm.* Usually donated, frozen sperm are used for therapeutic insemination in couples with severe male factor infertility. Sometimes men who must undergo treatments, such as chemotherapy, radiotherapy, or surgery, that would destroy their capacity to produce sperm also opt to freeze sperm for later procreation. Ironically, the introduction of ICSI is reducing the reliance on donor sperm because infertile men with poor sperm production are now able to father children. (For more information on donor sperm see Chapter 8.)

▪ *Frozen embryos.* About 15 percent of all ART cycles in 1996 used frozen embryos. In general, frozen embryos don't work as well as fresh ones. But many choose this option for a variety of reasons, including physical, emotional, financial, and philosophical.

Based on the 1996 data on frozen embryos, the live birth rate per thaw was 16.0 percent, and per transfer was a slightly higher 16.6 percent. In contrast, the live birth rate from fresh embryos per transfer was 27.9 percent. (One point to keep in mind is that, in general, fewer frozen than fresh embryos are transferred per cycle. This may bring the success rate down.)

- *Frozen eggs.* One of the most exciting advances in ARTs in recent years has been the successful freezing and thawing of human eggs. These advances in cryopreservation are helping a growing number of women—particularly older ones—conceive and give birth to healthy babies. At this point, there have been only a couple of successes, so the technique must still be considered investigational.

The ARTs represent a major step forward in the treatment of infertility from all causes. But the issues involved in deciding to enter an ARTs program are many, and they deserve your careful consideration. In the next chapter we take up some of those issues, and provide you with information that will help you evaluate programs to find the one that's right for you.

Just the facts

- IVF success rates have so improved that GIFT, and particularly ZIFT and TET, are used less and less frequently.

- ICSI is a highly successful and relatively new ART that is helping men with very low sperm counts father children.

- Assisted hatching seems to be helping to improve implantation rates.

GET THE SCOOP ON...
Selecting the best ART for you ▪ Funding the
ARTs ▪ Success rates in the ARTs

Chapter 8

Considering the ARTs

Now that you know what the ARTs are there are some things you and your partner should think about before looking for a specific program.

Making the decision to undergo ART is a momentous one. The success rates for ARTs are at least equal to the odds for an average, fertile couple to conceive in any given month. Just as the chances of conceiving from unprotected sexual intercourse does not increase with each month that a couple attempts to get pregnant, the probability doesn't increase with ART.

ART, emotions, and ethics

So making the decision to go with the ARTs is not easy. It's difficult to enter into an expensive treatment that has a much greater chance of failure than success. But if this might be your only chance of pregnancy, you need to think long and hard about the emotional and physical, as well as the financial, toll of these treatments. There are no guarantees in the ARTs; no guarantee that viable eggs will be

❝

Infertility treatments can be very seductive. There's always the promise that this month is different, this is the right month: the timing is better, the sonograms look better, you're feeling better this month than the last. You can loose your perspective very easily.
—Millie, who ultimately adopted two children

❞

harvested or fertilized, and no guarantee that a fertilized egg will divide properly, or that an embryo will implant and pregnancy will take place.

For these reasons, pursuing the ARTs can be an emotional roller coaster for many couples. They must deal with the possibility that these methods are the last resort in their attempt to have their own biological children. Then there is the waiting at nearly every step in these methods: Waiting to see if follicles will develop. Waiting to see if they can be retrieved. Waiting to see if they become fertilized. Waiting to see if they develop properly. Waiting to see if there are embryos to be transferred. Waiting to see if they implant. Waiting to see if the pregnancy continues. And, perhaps, even waiting for a coveted place in the ARTs program of your choice in the first place. It's no wonder that most couples going through the ARTs feel anxious, fearful, and, unfortunately for so many, disappointed, even devastated and angry.

These feelings are often exacerbated by the side effects of the fertility drugs that play a large role in any ART therapy. These drugs can throw your emotions into turmoil. (See Chapter 5 for more information on the side effects of hormonal therapy.)

Besides these considerations, you and your partner must be comfortable with the philosophical and theological issues that are bound to come up during these treatments. You may have faced some of these already during diagnosis, but now that you're going ahead with the decision to try the ARTs, they become far less theoretical. And the ARTs have their own set of ethical considerations, as well.

Here are some questions you and your partner should consider before looking into a specific ARTs program:

- What are our chances of pregnancy with other traditional therapies?
- Do we have time to wait for these other treatments to work?
- Are we comfortable with the idea of conception outside the uterus?
- Do we want to freeze embryos?
- What do we do with unused frozen embryos?
- How do we feel about donor sperm? Donor egg? (See Chapter 9 for a discussion on third-party reproduction.)
- What do we do if I become pregnant with triplets or quadruplets?
- When will we stop these treatments?

Choosing an ARTs program

Once you've talked about the "big issues" surrounding the ARTs, the next step is to find a program that's right for you. Much of the advice about finding the right doctor described in Chapter 3 of this *Unofficial Guide* also applies to finding the right ART program. Keep in mind several of the same key elements we discussed back in Chapter 3: Competency, compatibility, and convenience are critical. Because ARTs are expensive, cost is an important consideration, as well.

Competency is key

When evaluating whether a program's right for you, there are two critical sources of information that you should be sure to contact. The first is the *American Society for Reproductive Medicine (ASRM)*,

Timesaver
If you're seriously thinking about an in vitro fertilization (IVF) program, don't limit yourself to one program's wait list. Explore several. Your turn may pop up sooner at one program than another.

formerly the American Fertility Society. Call them for their guidelines on ART programs. Use these guidelines as a starting point to gather details about a program or programs. You'll learn a great deal about how these treatments should be performed and who they help the most—information that will help you select the most appropriate treatment program for you.

The second source to contact is the *Society for Assisted Reproductive Technology (SART)*, a specialty branch of ASRM, which focuses on high-tech clinical and research issues. Since 1993, SART has been gathering and publishing information on ART programs in the United States and Canada. In fact, any program that's a SART member and performs at least forty treatment cycles per year *must* report results to the SART Registry. Interestingly, a few of the finest programs in the country do not belong to SART. So, be prepared to do your homework. You can obtain a copy of that information directly from SART. (See Appendix B for details on how to contact ASRM and SART.)

Next start calling individual programs for their patient information packets. Most of them will have professionally produced educational materials ready to mail off to you upon request. Just don't be fooled by flashy, glitzy promotional brochures.

Armed with these patient information packets you can begin asking the hard questions about individual programs. At a minimum, you should ask the following:

- Are you part of the SART Registry?
- What procedures do you do? (IVF? GIFT? ZIFT? Sperm/egg micromanipulation? Donor sperm/egg? Cryopreservation?)

Watch Out!
It's probably a good idea to consider a program that does more than 100 cycles each year. Remember, if you go to a program that does less, you might not be getting as much experience. But, if you go for one that does more, you may just become a number.

- What are your success rates? (See the discussion about interpreting success rate statistics later in this chapter.)

Check that the program has on-site labs and monitoring equipment and that they are well staffed. The purpose of the fertility drugs used in ART treatments is to get you ovulating and to increase the number of eggs available for retrieval. Monitoring equipment must be on site not only to look for the right time to get those eggs, but to be certain that you don't develop ovarian hyperstimulation syndrome.

Compatibility concerns

You'll be spending a lot of time—and money—with these programs, to say nothing of the emotional energy you'll be expending. So it's important that you make certain that the program has a good support team of doctors, nurses, social workers, counselors, other patients, and even financial advisors who can help you every step of the way, cycle through cycle of therapy. Again, here are a few basic questions to ask:

- Do I have a choice of doctors?
- How experienced are your doctors? Your embroyologist?
- Will I be assigned to one or more doctors? Nurses? A Team?
- What counseling services are available?
- Is there the option of both individual *and* group counseling?

Convenience counts

ARTs require a great deal of time. If you've gone through ovulation induction, you may already have

Bright Idea
Get to know the people who are treating you. Key in on one or two. It'll help to hear test results—whether good or bad—from a familiar voice. And try to have someone with you when you call for test results. It might make hearing disappointing news a little easier and make sharing good news even more joyous!

a good idea of what's involved. So, ask, "How much time is involved in ART cycles?" "How much work will I miss?" If you must travel a distance to a program, ask, "What accommodations are nearby?" "Does the program help arrange lodging?"

Check out the availability of staff and technicians. Your doctor and clinic *should* have weekend and holiday hours. If you ovulate near the weekend they must be ready to retrieve your eggs.

Cost considerations

ARTs are very expensive. Just one IVF cycle complete with ovulation induction can cost upwards of $10,000. And if you go for more than one attempt, the costs can become prohibitive. Remember that cycles are sometimes cancelled. So ask:

- How much does an initial consultation cost? A screening?

- What does each drug and procedure (retrievals, inseminations, cryopreservation, transfer) cost?

- Do I pay in advance?

- What payment methods do you accept?

- Is a financial office/manager available to help submit bills?

This last point is very important—insurance coverage of ARTs is still a difficult issue, and good financial advice on how to fund your treatments will be extremely important.

Defining ART success

When gathering information about a program's success, you'll need to understand what the numbers they provide you actually mean. Ask each program to explain how they calculate their success rates and to define the terms they use. If you don't understand, ask again—and again, if necessary—until you do.

Remember, ART is a multi-step process. Success rates are reported based on the individual steps we mentioned in Chapter 7—ovulation induction, retrieval, fertilization, embryo transfer, and implantation. But not everyone goes through all the steps. For example, just because you start a treatment cycle it doesn't mean that you'll ovulate, or that eggs will be retrieved or fertilized, or that embryos will form, survive, and be transferred, let alone implanted and produce a live birth.

When questioning the program, try to get a sense of their philosophy about procedures. For example, do they transfer only the very best quality embryos or do they transfer borderline ones. The answer may give you insight into whether they are more concerned about doing procedures or about the outcome.

Also, when comparing one program's successes with that of another, make certain you're comparing apples with apples. For example, if you're looking at two program's reported success rates for embryo transfer, make sure both programs were transferring the same number of embryos.

Interpreting success rates

Here are definitions of the three terms used most often to calculate or define ART success rates. Become familiar with them so that you can understand the claims each program makes for itself.

- **Biochemical pregnancy.** In essence, this is an early positive pregnancy blood test result that is relatively common after any type of IVF procedure, as it would be in an unassisted conception. Unfortunately, as also occurs in

Timesaver
Some ART programs close for vacations—sometimes lasting a month or more. When looking at programs, be sure to check their year-long calendar. Make sure their schedule fits into yours.

Unofficially...
When comparing one program's success rate with another's, keep in mind that some programs take on the harder cases, so their success rates might be misleadingly lower.

unassisted conception, many of these biochemical pregnancies don't go on to produce a baby. Don't be fooled by a high biochemical pregnancy rate. It's really not telling you much about how good the program is.

■ **Gestational sac pregnancy.** Some programs use ultrasound examination to look for a gestational sac, the fluid-filled structure surrounding an embryo in the uterine cavity early in a pregnancy, and call that a pregnancy. Unfortunately, not all of these pregnancies will go on to produce a baby.

■ **Clinical pregnancy.** A clinical pregnancy is one in which the pregnancy hormone hCG level has continued to rise and a gestational sac, a fetal pole, and a fetal heart are detected during ultrasound examination. This usually occurs during week five or six. Most programs define success in terms of clinical pregnancy per treatment cycle. This figure would include everyone who begins taking fertility drugs whether or not eggs have been retrieved, fertilized, or embryos transferred. Other programs calculate success in more conservative terms—they give the clinical pregnancy rate based on embryos actually transferred.

It's very important for you to get an idea of how many women begin treatment and then go on to retrievals. It'll be an indication of how good a program's ovulation induction protocols are. But remember, clinical pregnancies are still *early* pregnancies and miscarriages and ectopic pregnancies do occur. Another factor to consider is cryopreservation. A single ovulation cycle might actually be responsible for a pregnancy realized after the second or third attempt at embryo transfer. This means that pregnancies from a single ovulation-induction cycle are increasing.

▪ **Take-home baby rate.** The single most important figure to look at is the live-birth rate, sometimes called the take-home baby rate. After all, the ultimate goal of any infertility treatment is the birth of a live baby. This is the only true indication of a program's success. This rate should reflect the number of *women* who take babies home, not the number of *babies* brought home. If one woman walks out of the program with three babies, it's still only one success story— not three.

ART program success rates

Under Federal law (specifically, the Fertility Clinic Success Rate and Certification Act of 1992), the 300 centers offering ARTs *must* report their results. The second overall report, based on collated results from individual clinics, is co-authored by the Centers for Disease Control and Prevention (CDC) in Atlanta, ASRM, SART, and RESOLVE (the patient advocacy group). It was issued in February 1998 and was based on 1996 data. Most fertility experts agree that 1999 results, which will not be calculated for several years, will continue to show a steady improvement in success rates. According to the newest report, over 64,000 ART treatment cycles were performed, resulting in nearly 21,000 babies.

In vitro fertilization continues to be the most commonly performed ART procedure. Although they are used far less frequently, GIFT and ZIFT have shown slightly higher live birth rates per retrieval than IVF. As we mentioned earlier, one explanation may be that women undergoing GIFT and ZIFT have healthier reproductive systems to start with. (See Table 8.1: ART Success Rates 1996).

The likelihood of pregnancy in an ART cycle is between 9 percent and 39 percent, depending on the woman's age, the quality of the man's sperm, and the technique. When the couple's own fresh eggs and sperm were used, the success rate reported was 22.6 percent live births per cycle started and 26.2 percent live births per retrieval.

Although ICSI has only been used since the early 1990s, 30 percent of all the ART cycles initiated in 1996 incorporated this new technology. In fact, ICSI has one of the highest success rates—27.8 percent live births per retrieval—of any ART reported in the study.

TABLE 8.1: ART SUCCESS RATES: FOR COUPLES USING THEIR OWN FRESH EGGS AND SPERM (1996)

Procedure	Live Births Per Retrieval	How Often Used
IVF	25.9%	71%
GIFT	28.7%	5%
ZIFT	30.3%	2%
ICSI	27.8%	30%

Source: *The American Society for Reproductive Medicine*

Unofficially... Unfortunately, collecting and freezing several sperm samples doesn't much help to improve sperm concentrations. Somehow, sperm from men with an infertility problem doesn't seem to freeze and thaw as well as sperm from fertile men.

Frozen embryos don't do quite as well as fresh ones. But an attempt at frozen embryo transfer has the advantage of reducing the number of ovulation induction cycles you need to undergo. In 1996 nearly 9,300 cycles involved embryos that had been frozen by a couple in a previous cycle.

When fresh embryos were transferred, the live birth rate per transfer was 27.9 percent. When the couple's own previously frozen embryos, which doctors call nondonated frozen embryos, were used, the live birth rate per thaw was 16.0 percent and the live birth rate per transfer was slightly a higher— 16.6 percent. It's important to keep in mind that between half to three quarters of frozen embryos do not survive thawing.

Embryos from donated eggs do well. Of the 5,162 cycles involving embryos formed from donated eggs, the live birth rate per transfer was approximately 39.0 percent. (See Chapter 9 for more information on third-party reproduction.) Current data indicate the rate may be as high as 50 percent.

How often should you try?

Once you've made the decision to undergo an ART, one of the next hardest decisions is how many times you should try. Obviously, the answers are not just to be found in statistics, but some recent data compiled by the ASRM/SART might help you make some decisions.

In a study based on older data, ASRM/SART looked at the IVF success rates of fifty-four fertility treatment programs and found no significant decrease in the success rates for the second and third attempts. In their review of more than 4,000 cycles of egg retrieval, they found that success rates remained almost equal for the first two treatment cycles, then declined only modestly in the third.

It wasn't until the fourth attempt that both pregnancy and delivery rates began to decline significantly. It seems probable that IVF simply wasn't going to work for some of these couples, no matter how many times they tried. So if IVF is likely to be successful, you should know within two or three tries.

Bright Idea
Before you go for a procedure—no matter how simple, or how little anesthesia or sedation you're given—bring someone with you. At the very least you will receive emotional support. But a companion is critical in helping when you leave the center. Your doctor will probably advise you not to drive, and you may not be very steady on your feet.

Old age or old eggs?

Once again, it's worth repeating: the chance of conception and ongoing pregnancy decreases as a woman gets older, whether or not she has a fertility problem and regardless of the treatment.

There are many reasons why older age adversely affects a woman's fertility. Besides medical conditions that can worsen with time, older ovaries become resistant to natural and drug-induced hormonal stimulation. Fewer and fewer follicles are produced and FSH levels rise. Estrogen and progesterone levels decline, causing menstrual irregularities and making the uterus less receptive to pregnancy. Finally, older fertilized eggs are less likely than younger eggs to develop normally.

Today, more and more older women are undergoing ART procedures. (Table 8.2 shows the increase in the last decade in the number of IVF attempts in older women.) And ARTs are being tried early in the course of their treatment.

But what age counts more, the age of the woman or the age of her eggs? According to 1996 data, women in older age groups have a better chance of having a baby if they use donor eggs than if they use their own. Success rates declined steadily after age 30—to nearly zero for women age forty-six using their own eggs. Women older than thirty-one years of age tended to have much better luck using donor eggs.

TABLE 8.2: ART REGISTRY RESULTS OF IVF IN WOMEN OVER FORTY

Year	Number of Embryos Transferred	Clinical Pregnancies per Embryo Transfer	Deliveries
1988	198	20(10%)	8(4%)
1990	350	8(11%)	23(7%)
1993	3,482	526(15%)	333(10%)

Still, the overwhelming majority of women who underwent ART procedures—three-quarters of them—were between thirty and forty years of age. Very few women younger than twenty-five used ART. And very few women older than forty-five undergo ART with their own eggs.

Not surprisingly, women thirty-four years old or younger had the best success rate—a steady 25 percent. This figure dropped as women got older. If eggs from a young, fertile donor are used, however, your age doesn't have much influence on the outcome. A somewhat older review has shown that delivery rates are high (30 to 50 percent per cycle) and miscarriages and chromosomal abnormalities are low when eggs from a young donor are used.

Most large ART centers are reporting live birth rates above 30 percent per embryo transfer in women up to age fifty five who use donor eggs. Other statistics show that more than half of peri-menopausal women will deliver a live baby within three oocyte donation tries, and with more than 85 percent delivering by the fifth try. (This is a cumulative pregnancy rate.)

The short- and long-term risk considerations

Fortunately, the ARTs have proven to be very safe procedures. But whenever you undergo any medical treatment, there are always some risks, however slight, of which you must be aware. Some of these risks involve actual medical concerns; others deal with broader moral and ethical considerations. Some are short term, some are longer term. The short term risks are associated with drug therapy and the minimally to moderately invasive procedures employed:

Unofficially...
A new class of infertility? Perhaps. Today, scientists are learning more about how age affects conception and pregnancy, and donor eggs are being used more and more successfully. Doctors are now referring to what was once called age-related infertility as *reduced egg quality* or *declining ovarian function*. It's not how old a woman is that counts, it's how old her eggs are.

- **Drug therapy**. The major risk of fertility drugs is ovarian hyperstimulation syndrome. This serious side effect occurs in about 10 percent of women undergoing ovulation induction. (See Chapter 5 for more information about the risks and side effects of hormonal therapy.) Uncommon side effects include blood clots where the shots are given and local swelling, redness and pain.

- **Instrumentation**. As with almost any type of procedure, there is the risk of infection, bleeding that can sometimes be severe, or organ damage. Then there are the side effects from local or general anesthesia or sedation.

Long-term risks include multiple births, birth defects, chromosomal abnormalities, and cancer.

Multiple births

Most ART procedures rely on fertility drugs and statistics show that the likelihood of success increases if more than one embryo is transferred per treatment cycle. But with this comes concern about the possibility of multiple gestation and its inherent risks to both the fetuses and the mother. (See Chapter 5 for more information about fertility drugs and the risk of multiple births.)

In 1996, about half the babies born from ART procedures were single births, and about one quarter were twins. Less than 6 percent of the births were triplets or more. (The remaining clinical pregnancies did not result in live births.)

The ASRM encourages ART programs to develop their own guidelines on embryo transfers based on the types of procedures they do and patients they see. ASRM does, however, issue general guidelines on how many embryos should be transferred in an ART cycle.

But it's really a decision you and your partner need to make with your doctor's input. You should ask yourselves: "What will we do with the embryos not transferred in a particular cycle?" "How do we feel about conceiving more than one child?" "What if we're faced with the possibility of fetal reduction?" These are discussions better had before a situation develops that must be dealt with as a crisis or for a lifetime.

Deciding on the number of embryos to transfer depends on several factors, including the woman's age, the embryo quality, and the availability of frozen embryos.

Here's what the ASRM recommends:

- In young women who have good-quality embryos, no more than three embryos are usually transferred.

- In women age thirty-five to forty years, usually no more than four embryos are transferred.

- In older women and those who have had unsuccessful treatment cycles, up to five embryos may be transferred.

- If a donor egg is used, the donor's age should be considered in deciding how many embryos to transfer.

If you're undergoing GIFT, your doctor will probably add one more egg to each category in these guidelines.

Birth defects and chromosomal abnormalities
One concern has certainly been eliminated since the early days of IVF procedures: the risk of birth defects. A recent study has confirmed that IVF, and

Bright Idea
Ask any ART program you're exploring for their guidelines and rationale for embryo transfers. Compare them with those of the ASRM.

Bright Idea
Once you've talked over the maximum number of embryos to be transferred, be certain to sign an informed consent.

now ICSI, do not pose an increased risk of birth defects in children conceived by these high-tech procedures. A study of couples undergoing infertility treatments showed that children born from ICSI did not have more chromosomal abnormalities than children born through conventional IVF. In fact, children born from IVF with ICSI did not have more congenital birth defects than children born in the general population.

That being said, there have been recent reports that some infertile men who carry a specific Y chromosome defect responsible for their infertility may pass that defect onto their male offspring conceived through an ICSI procedure.

Ovarian cancer

Any drug should be used cautiously; fertility drugs are no exception. But the overwhelming majority of studies (all but a few, in fact) have found no connection between fertility drugs and cancer. Although some of the studies were flawed, the others did underscore the need for judicious use of fertility drugs. You should not take any fertility drugs for more than several months at a time and certainly for not more than a total of six months to a year. No one can say with absolute certainty that fertility drugs do or do not increase a woman's risk for ovarian or breast cancer. Trying to find a definitive answer is very difficult. Even in tens of thousands of women, only a few cases of these cancers would be expected to be found. (For more information on fertility drugs and cancer, see Chapter 5.)

Just the facts

- When evaluating ARTs programs, competency, compatibility, cost, and convenience are key.

- There are many different definitions of pregnancy that can be used in posting success rates: Make certain that you discover the live-birth rate when you evaluate a program.

- The Society for Assisted Reproductive Technology provides information on high-tech clinical and research issues, and can provide information on the ARTs programs you're considering.

Alternative Solutions for Today and Tomorrow

PART V

GET THE SCOOP ON...
Third-party reproduction methods ▪ Alternatives
to traditional surrogacy ▪ Pregnancy vs.
parenthood ▪ Telling family and friends ▪
The adoption option

Sometimes It Takes Three...or Even Four or More to Make a Baby

Chapter 9

A sperm. An egg. A baby. Sounds simple enough. But, as you well know, for infertile couples, making a baby is a long, difficult process. You may be at the point where you've exhausted many of the conventional options and assisted reproductive technologies (ARTs), which we discussed in Parts 3 and 4, respectively.

The good news is that reproductive medicine is expanding your options to have a child. In many instances, the baby will be completely genetically related to you; in some cases, partially; in others, not at all. For tens of thousands of couples it sometimes takes, as we will see, three to make a baby. And, depending on what factors are causing your infertility, it could take not just three, but four or even five. (See Table 9.1: How Many Make a Baby?)

TABLE 9.1. HOW MANY PEOPLE HELP TO MAKE YOUR BABY?

| | How Many? | The Couple | | | Donor Involvement | | | | |
| | | Husband's Role | Wife's Role | | | | | Carrier | |
		Sperm	Eggs	Uterus	Sperm	Eggs	Embryo	Eggs	Uterus
Normal Conception	2	✓	✓	✓					
Donor Sperm	3		✓	✓	✓				
Donor Eggs	3	✓		✓		✓			
Traditional Surrogacy	3	✓						✓	✓
Gestational Carrier (Donor Uterus)	3	✓	✓						✓
Donor Egg/Gestational Carrier	4	✓				✓			✓
Donor Embryo	4*			✓			✓		
Donor Egg/Donor Sperm	4*			✓	✓	✓			
Donor Sperm/Donor Egg/Gestational Carrier	5**				✓	✓			✓

* Genetically, the same as adoption, except the female partner carries and delivers the baby
** Genetically and biologically, the same as adoption

DEFINITIONS OF THIRD-PARTY REPRODUCTION

Sperm Donation: A fertile man donates his sperm to an infertile couple to be used to fertilize the female partner's egg.

Egg Donation: A fertile woman donates her eggs to an infertile couple to be fertilized by the male partner's sperm. The female partner carries the resulting embryo.

Embryo Donation: An infertile couple donates extra embryos produced through an IVF procedure to another infertile couple, the embroyos are carried by the infertile couple's female partner.

Traditional Surrogacy (Surrogate Mother): A woman agrees to be inseminated with the sperm from the male partner of an infertile couple and to carry the fetus to term for that couple.

Gestational Carrier (Donor Uterus or Gestational Surrogacy): A woman agrees to carry to term an embryo produced through an IVF procedure using an infertile couple's eggs and sperm.

Egg Donation/Gestational Carrier: A woman agrees to carry to term for an infertile couple an embryo produced through an IVF procedure using some other woman's donated eggs and the male partner's sperm.

Egg Donation/Sperm Donation: The female partner carries to term an embryo produced through an IVF procedure using donated sperm and donated eggs. (Similar to embryo donation, but the infertile couple does not use extra, unneeded embryos from another infertile couple.)

Egg Donation/Sperm Donation/Gestational Carrier: A woman agrees to carry to term for an infertile couple an embryo produced through an IVF procedure using some other woman's donated eggs and another man's donated sperm. (Similar to above, but the female partner does not carry the pregnancy.)

How? Through *third-party reproduction*. Third-party reproduction refers to the use of eggs, sperm, embryos, or a uterus that are donated by someone (donor) so that you (recipients) can become parents. In addition to the tens of thousands of married infertile couples who turn to third-party reproduction, it is a route sometimes taken by unmarried persons or gay couples who desire a family, as well as by infertile couples. It encompasses all the approaches we'll be discussing in this chapter, regardless of how many "parties" are involved in the process.

Considering third-party reproduction

As you see, the third-party reproduction options available to you are many—indeed, mind-boggling. In general, when considering third-party reproduction, you'll need to confront several important immediate and long-term issues. These issues become more complicated as the options themselves become more complex. They include, but are not limited to:

- Personal concerns
- Spousal reactions
- Marital effects
- Family and friends' reactions
- Confidentiality issues
- Religious prohibitions
- Legal issues
- Ethical considerations
- Financial costs

It's wise that you talk with your doctor, a counselor, clergy, and, most certainly, a lawyer about the medical, emotional, social, and legal ramifications of these options. Any legitimate donor program—

Unofficially...
Although no accurate records exist, an estimated 8,000 women are believed to have been contracted to be surrogate mothers.

whether totally private or connected with a fertility treatment center—will offer counseling services. In fact, most programs using third-party reproduction, particularly those involving eggs and embryos, require you, your partner, and the donor to undergo psychological evaluation. If needed, it's worthwhile to go outside the program for additional guidance, as well. You'll probably get a more impartial perspective. Think of it as getting a second opinion, something you're probably comfortable with after having gone through infertility testing and treatment.

We'll explore some of the major issues surrounding third-party reproduction mentioned above. But, these are, by far, not the only considerations you and your partner need to discuss. Joining a support group, such as RESOLVE, is a very helpful way to learn more about how these options might affect you, your partner, and your child today and tomorrow. You may have thought about some of these issues before, but when actually faced with the possibilities or after going through infertility diagnosis and other treatments, your views may have changed.

What are motherhood, fatherhood, and parenthood?

Whether we recognize it initially or not, at the heart of the matter of third-party reproduction are the questions: What is motherhood? What is fatherhood? What does it mean to become parents? These are important questions to discuss with your partner. The answers will help you separate the social role of parenthood from the biological and genetic contributions.

You and your partner should ask yourselves: Are we looking to become pregnant or are we looking

Bright Idea
Some donor programs require donors to be married or in stable relationships. Some do not. If your donor is in an on-going personal relationship, it's important to know how his or her partner feels about the process. Be sure the donor's partner has been psychologically evaluated and counseled, too.

to be parents? Are we enamored with the idea of pregnancy and the attention it may bring? Or, do we want to build our family? Remember, pregnancy lasts nine months, parenthood a lifetime.

If you decide not to pursue third-party reproduction or it's been unsuccessful, answering these questions may help you to think about another alternative solution—adoption. You might ultimately face the question: When do we stop trying to get pregnant and start trying to become parents? (See below for more information about adoption.)

Passing on genes

Closely related to the issues of motherhood and fatherhood are those of genetic and biologic link. It also may be helpful to understand what the terms "biologic" and "genetic" mean. These terms are confusing and many people use them interchangeably. But, they are not precisely the same.

As we mentioned earlier, depending on the third-party reproduction method, your child can be completely, partially, or not at all related genetically to you. Although not linked genetically to you, your child may be linked biologically to you. The same holds true for the donor.

For example, if you contract with a woman to carry an embryo from an IVF procedure using your sperm and eggs, you're genetically related to the child, but not biologically linked. If you carry an embryo donated by another infertile couple, you're not genetically linked to the child, but you are biologically linked.

In this *Unofficial Guide*, the term "genetically" related or linked refers to genes—from the sperm or eggs—being passed on to the child. The term "biologically" related or linked refers to some physiologic function—for example, the female partner or a donor carries and delivers the child. Again, how strong that genetic link is depends on what's donated. And, don't forget, the male partner's genetic link to the child gets stronger if, for example, his brother is the sperm donor. Likewise, the female partner's genetic link gets stronger if her sister is the egg donor.

Because third-party reproduction usually introduces another set of genes into your family gene pool, you should examine how you feel about having a child who is not completely genetically your own. Here, you might ask yourself, "How important is a genetic connection with my child?"

The ability to impregnate their wives and pass on their genes is a very important physical and emotional role for men. This may be because the process of impregnating a woman is the only bio logic, not to mention genetic, role they have in pregnancy and childbirth. They may, therefore, equate impregnation and genetic contribution as the only thing that makes them a father. If they can't "father" a child, they may feel that they have no other major contribution to make and fear that they will have no interest in or ability to bond with the child.

Women seem to have an easier time than men looking beyond the genetic and biologic connection, as well as seeking parenthood rather than pregnancy as their primary goal do. In fact, the term "to mother a child" refers to the social, *not* biological, connection. "To mother" means to care for, nurture and raise a child, and has nothing to do with being pregnant, giving birth, or any other biological function including breastfeeding. On the other hand, the term "to father a child" means to get a woman pregnant and, therefore, refers *only* to the biologic not social connection.

It's important to remember that being a parent is more than just contributing your genetic material. It involves getting up in the middle of the night for diaper changes, feedings, and fevers. It means being there for the long haul—long after the moment of conception has passed.

Coming to terms

Another issue to be dealt with is what to call those who donate their eggs, sperm, or bodies. For eggs and sperm, it's fairly simple—they're called *donors*. However, it can become a problem for both the recipients and the offspring when these donors are referred to as the *biologic* or *real* mothers and fathers.

The term *birthmother*, or worse still, *real mother*, is especially confusing. As we mentioned above, to mother means to care for a child. In most families, the woman is the primary person to fulfill that role.

To tell a child who is the result of third-party reproduction or adoption that some other woman is his or her real or biologic mother, one whom he or she has not met, is confusing at best, and possibly detrimental. In the view of many psychologists, a child's real mother and real father are those people who mother and father—that is, parent—that child. To imply they're not the child's real mother or father is not only untrue, it's an insult.

Unfortunately, these terms and labels can lead to or reinforce rejection many of these children sometimes feel and face. These children must sometimes deal with the fact that outsiders consider the people who they're closest to, the people who raised them, not their real parents.

Bright Idea
Just like the person who donates an egg or sperm is called a donor, the person who is pregnant with the child and gives birth could be called a bearer, birther, or birth person. These terms are much less emotionally charged than "birthmother."

To donate or to divide

Some couples fear that a donor will be an intrusion—emotionally, psychologically, or even legally—on themselves and their marriage. A big barrier to using sperm donors, for example, is its impact on both the male and female partners' self-image, self-esteem, and their marriage.

Men tend to equate fertility with virility. It's easy to understand then why some infertile men feel that resorting to a donor is unmanly. It poses a threat to some and can have a devastating effect on their egos. To some, then, the thought of another man's sperm getting their wives pregnant is totally unacceptable. They may feel that their partners are being unfaithful. Others feel their wives have been raped or assaulted.

A woman might also have difficulty accepting the idea of donor sperm. Some may feel that using donor sperm conveys unintentionally to their partners that they don't love them. They see it as betraying their spouses. After the experience, some women have also felt as though they were violated or attacked.

Using donor eggs can produce similar reactions in both partners. A man who encourages his partner to use donor eggs might give off the message that he doesn't really care about her as a person, but only as a mechanism to produce a baby. A woman may feel she's a failure if she doesn't have eggs. And, because largely older women are using donor eggs, some women may feel they're getting "old and decrepit."

Using a surrogate or gestational carrier can confound these feelings. Seeing another woman clearly pregnant from her partner's sperm can devastate an infertile woman's self-image. She may see herself as

Unofficially...
No anonymous sperm donor has been held legally responsible for his offspring. In fact, in 1968, the California Supreme Court ruled: "The anonymous donor of the sperm cannot be considered the 'natural father' as he is no more responsible for the use made of his sperm than is the donor of blood or a kidney."

less feminine and less desirable. She may see the surrogate as a threat to her marriage. Certainly, many couples—whether fertile or infertile—often fantasize about what it would be like when the wife is pregnant. A surrogate or gestational carrier can certainly be a big intrusion on that private dream.

Some doctors mix the donor's sperm with the male partner's on the off chance that the child will be genetically his. Some consider this practice questionable—psychologically. It might indicate that the couple—or at least the male partner—doesn't fully accept sperm donation. On the other hand, others feel that it's just a little wishful thinking, so what's the harm. Again, this is a decision that should be made by the couple with the help of a qualified infertility counselor.

In her book *In Pursuit of Pregnancy*, author Joan Liebmann-Smith, PhD, describes the experiences of a couple, Eric and Lisa, who decided to use donor sperm. Says Eric about what happened when he was with Lisa while she was being inseminated with donor sperm:

> I started to cry. I had a very difficult time with the thought of somebody going into my wife's body that wasn't me. That was my macho part again—I wasn't able to make Lisa pregnant, so I felt like a failure. But I was also crying about all that energy that went into this—a year-and-a-half's worth...and here I was in the room holding my wife, and she was trying to get pregnant and it wasn't by me! I really felt the loss right there.

Lisa also had trouble with the concept of accepting sperm from a man other than her husband:

A few days before the insemination I absolutely freaked. The idea of foreign sperm was *so* disgusting. And, I screamed at Eric, "How could you want me to do this?" Then I found out when I went to our support group that this feeling passes. I began to think of the donor sperm as medicine, and it clicked. I said, "OK. If it's medicine, it's all right."

Lisa became pregnant after her first attempt with donor sperm. Both she and Eric were ecstatic. Said Eric about their experiences with infertility and donor insemination,

When someone pulled the cord on me and put up a roadblock and said, "Stop! You can't do that!" We found alternatives. Taking those choices along the road and getting to where we are now has made me feel this amazing closeness to Lisa. This child that isn't even born yet has brought us a whole lot closer than we ever were. It's really a commitment to a relationship. It's really a commitment to life.

Family matters

Some couples find resistance when they discuss third-party reproduction options with relatives. The potential grandparents may feel they'll be cheated out of a "real" grandchild—one genetically linked to them. They may wonder about the future grandchild's genetic well-being. Fearing family objections, many couples don't discuss their decisions with family, at least at first.

Keep in mind that a genetic connection can be a mixed blessing. You have to accept the good with the bad. Many people are under the false assumption that they will only pass on their good genes, and never consider that their offspring may be

Unofficially...
More than 90 percent of physicians who treat infertility with sperm donation use anonymous sperm donors.

Watch Out!
Some religions do not allow the use of donated sperm. If you think your religion forbids or frowns upon a particular aspect of third-party reproduction, talk to your religious leader and your doctor. There are often ways to adhere to your religious principles and still use these methods.

more like their weird Uncle Harry than their beloved Aunt Harriet.

For some couples and their families, passing along genes also means passing along religion. Some religions, like Judaism, hold that the child's religion is passed to them from their genetic mother.

Legal considerations

The legal concerns surrounding third-party reproduction are many—well beyond the scope of this *Unofficial Guide.* (See Appendix C: Resources, for sources of detailed information on the legal ramifications of donor reproduction.) It's best to consult legal counsel to learn the laws governing various types of donor use.

Even in donor sperm insemination, the oldest and most widely used form of third-party reproduction, both you and your partner must sign a consent form before the procedure is performed. This consent usually waives your rights to learn the donor's identity. It states your responsibility to care for and support a child that may result from the procedure.

In other types of third-party reproduction, it gets more complicated and confusing. For example, some states forbid paying for eggs or embryos.

You'll need legal counseling to enter into traditional surrogacy, gestational carrier, and egg donation contracts, as well as finalizing parental rights. After all, in some types of third-party reproduction you must actually adopt the child. Laws are being written on these matters almost daily, so you must check.

You'll need to look into what identifying and medical information is available to you, your child,

and the donor(s), as well as when and how that
information might be accessed.

All these matters become even more critical if
you know the donor. The bottom line is that even if
you think you know the laws in your state, always
check with a lawyer familiar with these evolving
issues.

To know or not to know

One of the most important considerations in deciding to use a donor is whether you want to know the
donor and whether you want the donor to know
you. Like everything in third-party reproduction,
the options are many. Here are just a few:

- Total anonymity prevails. (Sometimes called
  closed or *anonymous* donation.) You don't know
  the donor; the donor doesn't know you. For
  decades, this is the way it's been in the majority
  of donor sperm uses. You get a profile of the
  donor, maybe a photograph, but little more.

- Partial anonymity is maintained. You don't
  know who the donor is; the donor doesn't know
  you. But, you have limited contact, like speaking
  on the telephone. This is an option sometimes
  used when choosing an egg donor to help you
  feel more comfortable in your choice.

- Not anonymous, because some information is
  given. You both meet each other, but no identifying information is exchanged. This, too,
  sometimes happens with donor eggs.

- Open. You both meet and know about each
  other. This is the situation when arranging traditional surrogacy or for a gestational carrier.
  It's sometimes the arrangement that happens
  with egg donation.

MoneySaver
When contem-
plating tradi-
tional surrogacy
or using a gesta-
tional carrier,
calculate in the
potential hidden
costs: pregnancy
and delivery
complications,
such as a C-
section or mis-
carriage and
after care;
selective reduc-
tion for multiple
fetuses; and
amniocentesis.

▪ Known. This is the situation when the donor is someone you already know, like a family member or friend.

Each option has its pros and cons. In any type of third-party reproduction, you'll get—at the very minimum—a profile of the donor. It will describe the donor's medical history, as well as physical and intellectual characteristics. If you get to talk or meet the donor you can assess these attributes and qualifications yourself. Of course, no matter whether the donor is well known to you or anonymous, he or she can have financial rather than altruistic motives.

While choosing a friend or relative to be a donor may bring the parties involved closer, it can also cause problems. There can be disputes over child-rearing, contact with the child, and even custody. If the donor remains totally anonymous, there's little fear of donor interference in yours and your child's lives. After all, you may choose third-party reproduction, but you probably don't want third-party parenting.

When the donor has a face

As you've seen, dealing with a known donor can be complex. The more difficult aspects—emotional, as well as legal—of third-party reproduction come when the party doing the donating is contributing more than impersonal sperm and eggs. The issues may become a little more complicated when an infertile couple offers an unneeded embryo. Moreover, when a woman is offering her uterus to carry a child intended for you, the decision, the process, and its ramifications become highly complicated.

This can't be stressed enough: If you're contemplating third-party reproduction, but particularly,

Watch Out!
If you choose a brother or sister as a donor, you may confront sibling rivalry. One sibling may feel superior or inferior to the other. Past competitions between brothers or sisters may resurface.

when you're thinking about using a surrogate or gestational carrier, it's imperative that you seek counseling from trained professionals. These include both psychological counselors and lawyers.

Bright Idea
Be certain to discuss with a prospective surrogate your views on when and how an amniocentesis should be done and how you feel about pregnancy termination or fetal reduction.

You'll need to hire a lawyer who is knowledgeable and experienced in this highly complex area of family law and reproductive medicine. Some states accept some types of surrogacy, others don't. In fact, the practice is criminal in some states. Some states don't have any specific laws regarding surrogacy, which leaves you open to all sorts of difficulties down the road. Some states don't enforce laws they already have, which can also be a problem. Last, laws are changing almost daily.

There's growing concern over how donors will react after their donation. In the decades since donor sperm has been in use, little attention has been given to the long-term effect of sperm donation on the donor. Today, the increasing use of donor eggs is, however, bringing attention to the social and psychological effects of donation on the donor. Some women who at first felt altruistic about their egg donations have later expressed regret. They feel that they've somehow abandoned a child of theirs. Because many egg donors have had other children, they sometimes express sorrow at having given up a sibling of their other children.

If you're thinking about using donor sperm or eggs, this is something you and your partner should talk about, as well. After all, your child may, indeed, have half-brothers and half-sisters who they might later want to know. This need to know might be fueled if a medical situation arises in which a matched organ donor is needed. Then, of course, there is also the issue of a donor's "children" meeting, mating, and marrying inadvertently one day.

A recent survey of about a dozen women who served as surrogates a decade or so ago found they had no regrets about their decisions. But, many were disappointed that they weren't able to maintain contact with the infertile couple and child—although promised. Indeed, some felt betrayed that contact had been abruptly severed either right after the births or later. Some women in the survey do maintain consistent or occasional contact with the families.

In that same small Midwest study, researchers found that about one quarter of the women who had served as surrogates did so again, once or twice more.

To tell or not to tell

Ultimately, all couples choosing a third-party reproduction method face two important decisions. The first is what to tell their family and friends. The second is what to tell their child. With the emergence of the use of donor embryos, in which neither partner is genetically related to the child, these decisions become more complicated.

Many couples conceive babies through donors without anyone except their doctors knowing it. They decide that more harm than good can come from telling family or friends. And, it really is nobody's business except the child's.

For many couples whose children were conceived through third-party reproduction, being faced with the inevitable question, "Where did I come from?" takes on an entirely new dimension. As society becomes more conscious of family history, these questions also take on expanded meaning. There is considerable evidence, however, that it's best to tell children of donors about their genetic fathers, and now, mothers, when they're old enough to understand. Most therapists who specialize in infertility believe that family secrets are always bad and can backfire. Secrecy, many psychologists believe, can only lead to shame.

When a child is born from a donated embryo or through the use of a surrogate or gestational carrier, the issues can become more complicated, as more and more people are involved in making a baby and they're more closely involved with an actual child.

Some couples liken the use of donor embryo as a type of adoption. Genetically, the child may not be linked to you, but biologically through gestation, he or she is.

If a known donor is used, all parties must agree going into the process what their future relationships with the child will be. But, even if all agree starting out, keeping the circumstances surrounding the conception secret depends on the donor's discretion. Certainly, the donor's psychological, social, and even fertility status might change and affect a previously agreed-upon plan.

Deciding who, what, and when to tell must be left ultimately, however, to the couple. Joining a support group and/or seeking counseling from someone who specializes in the unique social and psychological issues surrounding third-party reproduction is imperative. After grappling with these issues most couples do come to a satisfactory decision.

As you can see many of these later options, which involve donor embryos and donor sperm/ donor eggs/donor uteri, raise issues that make them seem very much like adoption—an option that many couples ultimately choose.

Timesaver
If you're thinking
of private adop-
tion, you can
speed up the
process by send-
ing a letter or
e-mail about
your quest for a
baby to everyone
in your address
book. Be sure to
include all doc-
tors and lawyers.

The adoption option

If you decide not to use a donor or surrogate, or you have used a third-party solution unsuccessfully, you may want to consider what is actually another form of third-party reproduction—adoption. It's not something you think about right away. But after months or years of not conceiving, adoption usually becomes a real alternative to consider. Often, one spouse comes to this conclusion, however, before the other; more often than not, it's the female partner. Adoption is, perhaps, the most emotionally charged issue infertile couples face.

Losing the chance to have a genetic connection to a child is very difficult for most couples to accept. Most look forward to having children that resemble themselves and their families. And, as we mentioned earlier, many unrealistically think of children as a way of passing on positive family traits, as well as the family name. What they tend to forget about are all those skeletons in the family closet.

When considering adoption, it's a good idea to discuss with your spouse how each of you feels about having—or not having—a genetic connection to a child. Reread the section earlier in this chapter about passing on genes. You should ask yourselves, "Could we love a child not related to us?" If the answer is, "Yes!" or "Maybe," it may be time to start looking more seriously at the adoption option. If the answer is, "No," than adoption is probably not right for you—at least, not at this point. As Claire, a thirty-eight-year-old writer, put it:

> I know some people might be offended by this—and I'm certainly not equating the two—but when I ask myself if I could love a child not genetically related to me, I think about my dog.

I love that dog and would do anything for her. I would be devastated if anything ever happened to her. And she's not biologically related to me—or any human for that matter! If I could get that attached to my dog, of course, I would fall in love with my child.

As we said, women are usually more open to adoption, as well as the other third-party solutions, than men are. They often think about the possibility of adoption well before their partners even consider it a viable option. One reason: because women undergoing infertility treatment usually go through more both physically and emotionally than men; it might be somewhat easier for them to give up the idea of having a biological child.

On the other hand, some couples want to make it unmistakably clear to others that their child is adopted, so that there's no confusion in anyone's mind. Because of this, they choose to adopt a child from another race. This pretty much eliminates the embarrassing situation of people commenting on whom the child does or does not resemble.

Opposition to adoption

Remember, the decision to adopt is a very personal one, and it's not for everybody. If you or your partner feels strongly that adoption is not for you, it's better to realize that sooner than later. Some men—and women—are adamantly opposed to adoption and refuse to even discuss the issue. One woman said her husband was opposed to the idea because he didn't want "anybody else's trash." Others are opposed to adoption because they can't be guaranteed a normal, healthy child. One man told his wife, "If we can't have our own children, I don't want anybody else's children. And besides, there are no healthy, normal, intellectually curious, babies up for adoption anyway."

Most of us assume that we'll produce healthy, beautiful, intelligent children. But, keep in mind, we can't be assured a "perfect" child, even if we undergo pre-conception genetic testing and amniocentesis. Not every genetic, medical, or physical defect can be screened for. And, you can't rule out psychological problems prenatally. Your best traits, therefore, may not be passed on to your offspring.

It's not just concern about the adopted children that prevents some from wanting to adopt. For those men who see infertility as a reflection on their masculinity, adoption is extremely stigmatizing. It's proof positive to the outside world that they could not get their wives pregnant. Once they adopt, they can no longer pretend that they were childless by choice.

Adoption also represents giving up to some couples. But, remember, adoption is really just an alternative way of building a family. Here's how one woman described how her first reaction to adoption as "the ultimate failure" changed over time: "After about six months, adoption shifted to something one could possibly do and still try to get pregnant. Then, when I decided it wasn't worth trying to conceive any more, adoption became the *only* option."

If you decide to start pursuing adoption, remember that this decision is not written in stone—at least, not yet. The good news about adoption is you can change your mind until the papers are signed. The bad news is the pregnant woman can also change her mind.

Misconceptions about adoption

If you're still undecided and ambivalent about adoption, you and your partner might try writing down

Bright Idea
If you're considering adoption, use a lawyer who specializes in adoption. Adoption lawyers are not only the most qualified to help you with adoption, but also because they're on the front lines, they often hear about pregnant women who need to put their babies up for adoption.

what each of you sees as the pros and cons of adoption. Then, compare notes. It may also help to look at two of the common myths about adoption.

■ *If I adopt, I'll get pregnant.* This is one of the most persistent—and annoying—myths about adoption. Adoption guarantees you a baby, not a pregnancy. Studies, in fact, have shown that the number of infertile women who conceive after adoption is the same as the number who pursue other options. One reason the myth persists is that you're unlikely to hear anecdotes about someone's friend who adopts and *doesn't* get pregnant—it doesn't make very interesting cocktail party conversation. So, if you're considering adopting because you think it may lead to a pregnancy, you're probably adopting for the wrong reasons and setting yourself up for disappointment.

■ *There are no healthy newborns of my own race available for adoption.* This is also untrue. There are many healthy newborns of all races available through agencies, private adoption, and foreign adoption. You will find more information about these sources of adoption in the resource section of this book.

Further considerations

Deciding to adopt is just the beginning of the decision-making process. Here are some of other adoption-related issues you may confront:

■ Should you adopt through an agency or pursue private adoption?

■ Should you look into foreign adoption? If so, which countries?

■ Should you adopt a child of another race?

- Should you adopt an infant or an older child?

- Should you adopt a handicapped child?

- Should you have an open adoption and meet the woman who gave birth to your child? If so, should you have an ongoing relationship with her?

To help you address these issues and answer these questions, we have listed many excellent books on adoption and other adoption resources in the appendix of this book. Like infertility treatment, you need to take control of the situation and learn all you can about your various options. It will take time, effort, and a lot of research. But, the payoff is finally having your longed-for child. In fact, most couples can find the type of child they want to adopt within a few years at most.

While adoption isn't a cure for infertility, it's certainly a cure for childlessness, and the pain it causes. Adoption helps you put infertility behind you while opening up a whole new world of parenthood, as this woman happily discovered:

I really feel better at this point having stopped (infertility treatments), because we really feel we've done all we could do. Just this last week I began to have hope for the future. I'm forgetting the names of the fertility drugs. I don't know—or care—what day of the month it is. I used to know everything so well. I'm sure that's because we're so close to adoption—it's like something else to put our minds to.

I feel like I'm playing house, but I'm thrilled. I've been collecting cradles and rockers and little baths and I've been knitting little baby things. And, I don't even know when the baby is going to arrive. It could be next month. It could be the summer. It could be the fall. But now I feel it's legitimate and reasonable to make plans, because we're going to have a baby!

Just the facts

- There are healthy newborn babies of all races available for adoption.

- Adoption is a path to a baby, not a pregnancy.

- Joining a support group can help you make an educated decision about third-party reproduction.

- The laws regarding third-party reproduction vary tremendously from state to state.

- Using known sperm or egg donors may increase the chances of legal complications and custody battles.

- Most experts agree that children of third-party reproduction should be told the truth about their origins.

GET THE SCOOP ON...
Sperm, egg, and embryo donation ▪ Surrogacy ▪
Choosing a program ▪ Screening donors

Chapter 10

Pursuing Third-Party Reproduction

In Chapter 9 we looked at the various third-party reproduction options available—and you may have decided one of these seems right for you. If so, the next step is to find the appropriate doctor and program to help you through the many medical, psychological, and legal steps involved in making the final decision and plans to use these approaches.

Many of the same principles we mentioned in Chapter 3 on finding a fertility specialist and in Chapter 7 on finding an ART program apply when looking into a third-party reproduction program. These are good places to start. The other prime resources for information about third-party reproductions in general and specific programs:

- RESOLVE
- The American Society for Reproductive Medicine (ASRM)
- Your current fertility specialist

Moneysaver
Besides medical
treatment, your
spouse and your
donor and/or
surrogate will
need to undergo
some psychologi-
cal counseling.
You'll also need
help with legal
documents. You'll
most likely save
both time and
money if you go
to a program
that provides all
these services.

Ultimately, the program you choose for help for
third-party reproduction depends on what your medical needs are, as well as what you're ready emotionally to pursue and what you can afford financially.

What third-party reproduction programs handle

For convenience, we can look at the third-party
reproduction options in two broad categories: *donor
gametes*, which are sperm, eggs, and embryos; and
surrogacy, which includes traditional surrogacy (surrogate mothers) and gestational carriers. How much
involvement you'll need from your infertility specialist, an ART program, or donor agency depends
on the third-party reproduction method you need.
Here's a brief rundown of the options:

- Sperm donations are used widely and can be
  handled routinely through many infertility specialists and centers. They might have their own
  sperm banks or have working relationships with
  one or more.

- Egg donations, which are fairly new, are handled medically through ART centers, which may
  or may not have a program in place to find a
  suitable donor for you. If they don't, egg donations can be arranged through private agencies.
  (See below for more information about private
  agencies.) As with sperm donation, you might
  have a relative or friend who agrees to donate
  her eggs.

- Embryo donations are only handled through
  ART programs. They have the frozen embryos
  on hand and they do the transfers. They should
  assist you and the donor in all the necessary
  paperwork, medical and legal.

- Surrogacy may involve some of these aspects, particularly in a permutation in which donor sperm, egg, or embryo is involved. There are agencies specially set up to match a surrogate or gestational carrier with an infertile couple. Some of these programs also provide services to find donor eggs. Even if you have a prospective surrogate in mind, these agencies can help with the legal paperwork.

How private agencies help

There are private agencies that will assist infertile couples in many of the steps surrounding third-party reproduction—in particular, egg donation and surrogacy arrangements. Their services vary. They may:

- Maintain donor lists

- Screen donors

- Intermediate between the donor and recipient

- Work with medical centers chosen by the donor or recipient

- Coordinate legal services for both the donor and recipient

- Arrange legal and medical appointments, travel arrangements, disbursement of fees

That agency should be set up to help coordinate the medical aspects of the donation (psychological testing; screening; and arrangements for ovulation induction, egg retrieval, in vitro fertilization [IVF], and embryo transfer), as well as draw up the legal contracts between you and the donor.

There are pros and cons to using private or independent third-party reproduction. If you go private, you have to coordinate all medical and legal aspects

Timesaver
Choose a donor or surrogate program that carefully screens donor applicants and re-tests them periodically. Besides giving a good indication of how committed a donor is, it saves time by insuring that there's an adequate pool of qualified donors or surrogates on hand when you need one.

of the donation. In addition, you'll be having contact with the donor and the donor with you. Working through an agency, though more expensive, covers many of these items, as well as allows the option of some anonymity—at least in the case of sperm and egg donations.

What to ask

The American Society for Reproductive Medicine (ASRM) has guidelines for gamate donation, including sperm, egg, and embryo. Be certain the donor sperm and egg clinic—whether physician-based, hospital-based, or commercial—is following ASRM guidelines for monitoring and testing donors. *The American Association of Tissue Banks (AATB)* has established standards for tissue banking, including tissues used in reproductive medicine. They inspect and accredit member banks, similar to what's done for blood banks or clinical laboratories. Check that they accredit the program, as well.

When you're thinking about egg, donor, or embryo donation, write or call for patient information packets from programs around the country. By comparing the services they offer, you'll get a good idea of what you should be asking.

Screening donors

In accordance with federal and state regulations all sperm and egg donors must be screened for genetic diseases, hepatitis B and C, sexually transmitted diseases, and HIV. (You can get a list of these tests from the ASRM or AATB.) Many banks also run other blood chemistry tests and tests for other genetic and infectious diseases. Many of these tests are based on an evaluation made by a clinical geneticist of a potential donor's risk of carrying medical and hereditary diseases. You probably want to make sure

Watch Out!
All sperm or egg donors must be screened for disease, including for HIV.

that all sperm donors are screened, for example, for cystic fibrosis carrier status. Other potential donors are screened, based on their genetic background, for breast and ovarian cancer (BRCA-1) gene mutations, Tay-Sachs disease, sickle cell anemia, and thalassemia. Depending on the test and the program, tests are done initially then every six months; some programs retest more frequently. In addition, if an egg donor is older than thirty-four years (anonymous or known egg donors are usually younger than thirty-four years, but you may have a relative or friend who is a little older), you should plan to have a prenatal test to be certain the fetus is developing normally.

Bright Idea
If you're thinking about using a donor sperm or eggs, be sure to discuss genetic counseling with your physician. It's important for you to know your risk status so that no inadvertent genetic disease is passed to a child that results from third-party reproduction.

HIV

Only frozen sperm that has been quarantined for at least six months can be donated through an anonymous program in this country. This allows donors to be re-tested for antibodies to HIV, the virus that causes AIDS, which may not develop or be detected for several months after a person's exposed to the virus.

In addition, some programs will perform more sophisticated HIV testing using *polymerase chain reaction (PCR)*. PCR can actually test for virus inside cells months before HIV antibodies are seen in blood or semen. Testing potential donors with this method can eliminate donors before specimens are procured.

Because freezing eggs is ostensibly experimental, screening egg donors for HIV is a problem. While the risk of HIV transmission is low, it nonetheless exists. The program should be screening potential donors for disease before they are accepted. Once accepted and chosen to be a donor, they should be re-tested. But, as we mentioned

before, it can take six months before HIV antibodies
are detectable. There's no way to guarantee that the
eggs retrieved today are from a donor who wasn't
exposed to HIV last week.

In unusual cases recipient couples decide to
have the donor eggs retrieved, fertilized in an IVF
procedure, and any embryos frozen. The donor can
be re-tested six months later, and, if given a clean
bill of health, the embryos are transferred.
Remember, frozen embryo transfers are not as successful as fresh ones.

Infectious diseases

ASRM guidelines require that donor embryos be
quarantined for at least six months so that the
potential donors can be tested for infectious diseases before the embryos are transferred to the
recipients. There are situations in which donor testing may not be possible: for example, in a post-
mortem donation. (An infertile couple may have
specified their willingness to have extra frozen
embryos donated upon the death of either or both
the them.)

Bright Idea
It's not only the
donor who
should be tested
for HIV. It's a
good idea to test
the donor's part-
ner and the
recipients and
their partners,
as well.

Physical characteristics

Most of these programs will provide you with patient
profiles that allow you to closely match the donor's
physical characteristics (such as eye color, and hair
color and texture), ethnic and racial background,
and even occupation, special interests, and skills,
with that of the male or female partner. To help you
pick a sperm donor that might offer the best chance
to have a child that resembles your family, some
sperm banks allow you to submit your picture. Their
staff will rank the resemblance of the donor's with
your photo and the characteristics you've outlined.

Other general questions

The decision to go with a gamete donor is not to be taken lightly. In addition to the above items, here are a few other important questions you might want to ask:

- Do your donors have children themselves?
- Do you limit how many times a donor's sperm or eggs will be used?
- If so, how many?
- Are these limits confined to specific geographic areas or do they apply nationally?
- Do you limit how many stimulation cycles a donor undergoes?
- If so, how many?
- If a successful pregnancy ensues, can we use sperm or eggs from the same donor for another pregnancy?

As you have learned, infertility treatment is not guaranteed to get you pregnant. Certainly, the same is true for third-party reproduction. So, you should also ask the service, "What are my costs and liabilities if no eggs are retrieved from the prospective donor?" "If eggs are retrieved, but we do not get pregnant, can we change donors?" "If so, how much will it cost?" If you use a gestational carrier, you'll have another series of questions, including: "If the gestational carrier fails to get pregnant, what are our options?" "What are our financial and legal responsibilities?"

You should also ask, "What happens if an amniocentesis test result comes out abnormal?" "Will the carrier have an abortion and, if so, who pays for it?" "Who is responsible if the child is born abnormal?" and "Who will raise and care for the child?"

TABLE 10.1: THIRD-PARTY REPRODUCTION: WHO IT HELPS

Third-Party Reproduction Option	What You Contribute	Who It Can Help
Sperm Donation	Female partner's eggs and uterus	**Male partner who:**
		Has severe sperm, ejaculatory, or immunological problems
		Has a non-reversible vasectomy
		Doesn't produce sperm because of cancer treatment
		Has an hereditary defect
		Has failed sperm aspiration
		Has failed ICSI
		Has unexplained infertility
Egg Donation	Male partner's sperm / female partner's uterus	**Female partner who:**
		Has no eggs
		Doesn't ovulate
		Is too old to have any useable eggs
		Doesn't have ovaries
		Had her ovarian function destroyed during cancer treatment
		Has premature ovarian failure
		Has an hereditary defect
		Has failed ART
		Has unexplained infertility

Embryo Donation	Female partner's uterus	**Male and female partners who:**
		Haven't been able to produce an embryo or have an embryo survive
		Have an hereditary defect
Traditional Surrogacy	Male partner's sperm	**Female partner who:**
		Has had repeated ectopic pregnancies
		Has had repeated miscarriages
		Doesn't have ovaries or functioning ovaries; doesn't have a uterus or functioning uterus
		Has a medical condition that makes pregnancy unwise or impossible
Gestational Carrier	Male partner's sperm / female partner's eggs	**Female partner who:**
		Has a uterus that doesn't accept an embryo implantation
		Has suffered repeated miscarriages
		Doesn't have a uterus
		Has a medical condition that makes pregnancy unadvisable
		Has unexplained infertility despite conventional treatments and ART

continues

Third-Party Reproduction Option	What You Contribute	Who It Helps
Egg Donation, Gestational Carrier	Male partner's sperm	**Female partner:**
		Doesn't have useable eggs and/or doesn't have uterus
		Has a uterus that hasn't accept an embryo implantation using donor eggs
Sperm Donation, Gestational Carrier	Female partner's egg	**Female partner:**
		Doesn't have useable eggs and uterus
		Male partner:
		Doesn't have useable sperm
		Both male and female partners:
		Have hereditary defects
Sperm and Egg Donation, Gestational Carrier		**Female partner:**
		Doesn't have useable eggs and/or uterus
		Male partner:
		Doesn't have useable sperm
		Both male and female partners:
		Have hereditary defects

Because traditional surrogacy or the use of gestational carriers pose their own unique set of concerns, you might ask: "What experience does your center have with gestational surrogacy?" "Do you have specially trained counselors in this area?" "What surrogacy contract experience does your legal staff have?"

If you're going to be using donated embryos, you should ask: "What is your success using frozen embryos?" Like any other type of third-party reproduction also ask: "What are the charges for embryo thawing, transfer, cycle coordination and documentation, and infectious disease screening of both recipients and donors?" You should also ask the program how the embryos themselves came to be. Ask: "Are these embryos the product of an infertile couples eggs and sperm, or were the eggs and/or sperm donated?" The program should document that all the appropriate screening was performed.

Sperm donation

Couples choose sperm donation in a variety of circumstances, but in every case, the problem is that the male partner can't contribute useable sperm. For example:

Scenario #1: John and Mary have been trying to conceive for three years. But John has severe male-factor infertility due to an ejaculatory duct obstruction from a past infection. He has undergone surgery and sperm aspiration, and Mary has undergone artificial insemination with John's sperm, as well as IVF with ICSI—all to no avail.

Scenario #2: Henry and Sally want children, but Henry's aunt and his brother both died in their forties from Huntington's disease, a rare, hereditary, degenerative disease which they didn't want to risk passing along.

The third-party reproduction solution in both cases would be to use donor sperm. John and Mary opted to use John's brother, Don, as a donor. However, because Henry has a 50% chance of passing the gene for Hungtington's disease on to his offspring, he and Sally decided to use anonymous donor sperm.

Sperm donation was the first and still the most commonly used third-party reproduction method. It's been an option for thousands of couples over the last six decades. It uses three people to make a baby: The man who donates his sperm and the infertile couple who uses it.

What to Expect: Donor sperm insemination is very similar to therapeutic insemination with husband's sperm (TIH), with a few exceptions. The donor's sperm must be collected and frozen for at least six months to allow the donor to be re-tested for communicable and deadly diseases.

Most often, donor inseminations are performed via *intrauterine insemination (IUI)*, which increases the chance of success. They can be used in ART procedures, as well.

The Pros:

- You pass along the female partner's genetic makeup to your child.

- The female partner has the chance to experience pregnancy and childbirth and the male partner has the opportunity to share in it.

- Even if you use an anonymous donor, you can usually pick some characteristics, like hair or eye color, with the hope that the child will look more like the both of you.

- It's one of the least invasive and safest solutions to male-factor infertility.

Unofficially...
The first widely covered third-party reproduction case occurred in 1934 when a woman from Long Island, New York, gave birth to twins after being inseminated with donor sperm. A *Newsweek* article of that day referred to the men who donated their sperm as "Ghost Fathers."

- Unless you tell, no one will know you've taken this route to conception.

The Cons:

- Your child gets half of his or her genes from someone other the male partner.

- If you don't know the donor, you don't really know their complete medical and family history.

- There's always a remote risk of infection even if donor and his sperm are carefully screened.

- As we mentioned earlier, using donor sperm can create marital conflicts.

Watch Out!
Even if the donor is a family member, it's imperative to wait the six months to have him re-tested for communicable diseases, such as AIDS, which may not be detectable in blood tests when first exposed.

Egg donation

As with sperm donation, the reasons for a couple to opt for turning to an egg donor can vary, but they all share a fundamental cause. The female partner can't contribute eggs.

Scenario # 1: Although Hannah is only thirty-one, she has experienced premature ovarian failure and no longer produces eggs. She is otherwise healthy and wants to experience pregnancy and childbirth, so she and her husband have decided to ask her sister, Donna, to be an egg donor. Donna, who has three children, readily agreed.

Scenario #2: Ellen married Sam when she was in her early forties. Although Sam has children from a previous marriage, they would like to have children together. Ellen, who still gets her period, has tried Clomid and Pergonal, but they haven't worked very well. They have decided to undergo IVF using eggs donated anonymously.

Using donor eggs is one of the newest advances in third-party reproduction. This is another example in which three people are involved in making a

Unofficially...
Although an egg
donor is tested
for medical,
genetic, and
communicable
diseases, there's
really no guaran-
tee that she
doesn't have the
virus that causes
AIDS. There are
lag times
between the
points a prospec-
tive donor signs
on, is accepted,
chosen by an
infertile couple
to be the donor,
and the time of
egg retrieval and
IVF. While the
chance of pass-
ing along HIV is
remote, it's still
not zero.

baby: The woman who donates the eggs and the infertile couple who receives them. For many couples, donor eggs have replaced the use of traditional surrogacy (surrogate mothers).

What to Expect: Eggs, which have been donated usually anonymously, but sometimes from a known donor, are fertilized through an ART method. The donor would most likely receive fertility drugs to increase the number of eggs available for fertilization and you'll receive hormones to prime your uterus for embryo implantation. Any extra embryos produced may be frozen for future transfer attempts.

Donor eggs are quite successful because they usually come from healthy, young women, who are likely to have healthy, young eggs. In fact, donor egg success rates are about the same for older women as ART is for younger women.

The Pros:

■ Your child is genetically related to the male partner.

■ You get to experience pregnancy and childbirth.

■ It's really the first time older and post-menopausal women have been able to have children.

■ Extra embryos may be frozen for future transfer attempts.

■ If both the fresh and the frozen embryo transfers are successful the children will be siblings genetically.

■ Unless you tell, no one outside the family will know you've taken this route to conception.

The Cons:

- Both the egg donor and recipient must take hormones to synchronize the egg donor's ovulation with the recipient's ability to implant an embryo. (Of course, if frozen embryos are used, timing needn't coincide.)

- This is costly. If an anonymous donor is used, there's a fee to find, screen, and match the donor with you. Then, there's compensation to the donor for her time and inconvenience. (Human eggs can't be sold in this country, but women do receive money for participation in the program and their expenses.)

- Because egg donation involves ART procedures, there are those expenses as well.

- There are, of course, legal fees and issues.

- If a known donor is used, there's a risk that the donor will be overly involved with the pregnancy and child, or may even sue for custody.

Embryo donation

If you and your partner haven't been able to produce fertilizable eggs or your fertilized eggs haven't divided properly for transfer, embryo donation is a further option to explore.

Scenario #1: Bill and Sarah both have fertility problems. They have undergone six IVF procedures, including two with ICS, but they haven't been able to produce a "good-quality" embryo for transfer. They've even had two cycles with donor eggs. Since all indications are that Sarah's uterus is fine, their doctor suggests they use embryos donated anonymously by an infertile couple at that ART center.

Moneysaver
Be sure to freeze any good quality embryos produced from donated eggs. This will reduce the cost of another round of fertility drugs for the donor. But, remember, success with frozen embryos isn't as good as with fresh embryos.

Scenario #2: Debbie and Ben both have infertility problems. She has elevated FSH levels, which indicate a diminished capacity to produce eggs. He has severe male factor infertility. They do, however, want to experience pregnancy and childbirth, so they opt to use donated embryos.

Embryo donation has become a viable option for infertile couples since the availability of IVF programs and cryopreservation. Infertile couples who become pregnant and no longer need their embryos are seeing this as a way of helping other infertile couples. This solution also involves four people: The infertile couple receiving the embryo and the infertile couple who donated the embryo.

What to Expect: The female partner will take hormones to prepare her uterus for embryo transfer, which is done during an IVF procedure.

The Pros:

▪ You get to experience pregnancy and childbirth.

The Cons:

▪ You and your partner are not genetically related to the child.

▪ You'll take some drugs to help prepare your uterus for embryo implantation.

▪ It's costly because of the drugs and procedures involved.

▪ You'll need legal counseling because laws governing embryo donation differ from state to state and you must have explicit prior approval from the donors to use the embryos.

Unofficially...
More than 1,000 babies have been born in the U.S. through egg donation.

Donor sperm/donor eggs

If neither partner has useable sperm or eggs, but the female partner does have a uterus that will probably accept an embryo implant and continue an on-going pregnancy, a third-party reproduction solution is the use of donor sperm to fertilize donor eggs via IVF.

Scenario #1: Karen and John are both forty. John had undergone treatment for testicular cancer when he was thirty, hadn't banked any sperm before therapy, and is now sterile. Karen no longer ovulates. They want to experience pregnancy and childbirth, but decide against using a donor embryo. They reason: "We don't want our child to have half-brothers or half-sisters she or he doesn't know. And, besides, it's risky. What if they want their children to know their half-siblings and track us down? And, if something happens to one of their children, would they try to gain custody of John Junior?" So they choose an anonymous sperm donor and an anonymous egg donor.

Here, four people are involved. The infertile couple, plus the man who donated the sperm, and the woman who donated the eggs. This is tantamount to using a donated embryo, except that the sperm and egg donors probably don't know each other and hadn't otherwise planned to produce an embryo.

What to Expect: The donor takes drugs to increase the number of eggs available for retrieval. You'll be given hormones to prepare your uterus to accept any embryos produced. This must be coordinated with the egg donor's ovulation.

The Pros:

- You get to experience pregnancy and childbirth.

- You eliminate the possibility that an infertile couple who no longer has a need for their embryos gets any second thoughts.

- Extra embryos produced may be frozen for future transfer attempts.

- If successful, you might try again using these extra frozen embryos. That would make the siblings genetically related.

The Cons:

- You're not genetically related to the child, unless you use a relative. Even then you're not totally related.

- This option involves an IVF procedure and preparation of your uterus for embryo transfer.

- Expensive because an IVF procedure is used and you must find two suitable donors.

Traditional surrogacy

One common infertility problem is that the female partner can't carry a pregnancy to term. The earliest, and one of the most controversial, third-party reproduction option to become available to couples in this situation was traditional surrogacy. This option involves three people: The infertile couple and the woman who carries the fetus.

Scenario #1: Desiree has premature ovarian failure, which means she doesn't produce eggs. Her husband, Don really wanted a child genetically related to at least one of them. Since his sperm were fine, the doctor recommended surrogacy, which was legal in their state. Through an agency recommended by their doctor, they found a woman they both liked who agreed to be a surrogate for $10,000.

Scenario #2: George and Martha married in their mid-forties. Since Martha wasn't ovulating, they tried egg donation, but each embryo transfer ended in a miscarriage. When their physician suggested traditional surrogacy, they rejected the idea

Unofficially...
Many agencies that arrange for surrogates or gestational carriers are calling these individuals host uteri or fertility assistants.

of using a stranger. They feared getting embroiled in a custody battle like Mary Beth Whitehead did over "Baby M." Instead, they asked Martha's younger sister, who already had three children, to be the surrogate and she agreed.

Before the advent of egg donation, you might have used this option if you couldn't produce eggs or your eggs couldn't be fertilized. Now the indications for traditional surrogates are narrower than they used to be. You might use this option if you can't continue a pregnancy long enough to deliver a viable fetus.

What to Expect: You'll contract with a woman to be therapeutically inseminated—usually in an IUI (intrauterine insemination) procedure—with the male partner's sperm and to carry that child to term. Her ovulation will be monitored to time the insemination with her fertile period, but more than one attempt might be necessary.

The Pros:

- The child inherits the male partner's genes. If a family member of the female partner becomes the surrogate, the child is genetically connected to that side of the family, as well.

- It's not medically invasive to any participant.

- You get to monitor the surrogate's medical progress throughout the pregnancy.

- You can pick the surrogate who gives birth to your child.

The Cons:

- The child gets half his or her genes from someone outside the family, unless the surrogate is related to the female partner.

Watch Out!
You pretty much have to trust your surrogate isn't going to have intercourse and get pregnant by someone else. Just because a woman you've contracted with to be a traditional surrogate passes a pregnancy test the day of the insemination with your sperm, doesn't mean she's isn't already pregnant with another man's child or that she hasn't contracted some disease.

■ It can be quite expensive because it involves
locating a suitable surrogate and paying her
legal fees and medical care.

Gestational carrier

Bright Idea
Just because
another woman
has actually
delivered your
child doesn't
mean you can't
breastfeed.
Groups, like the
La Leche League,
can help you
learn more about
induced lacta-
tion. Through
mechanical and,
sometimes,
hormonal stimu-
lation, most new
mothers can pro-
duce at least
some milk for
their babies.

There are cases where the female partner can produce perfectly viable eggs and the male partner's
sperm is healthy, but infertility remains an issue.
This can be the case if the female partner doesn't
have a uterus, or cannot carry a pregnancy to term.
In this situation, one option is to turn to a gestational carrier, which some prefer to call a donor
uterus. This is another option involving three
persons: The infertile couple and the woman who
carries and delivers the child.

Scenario #1: When Bob asked Carol to marry
him, she told him that she could never have children because she was born without a uterus. Bob
said he didn't care, they could always adopt. Around
the time they were ready to have children, Carol saw
a TV special about gestational carriers called, "A
Womb for Rent." She and Bob decided that this
would be a great solution for them since the child
would be genetically theirs. Their doctor referred
them to an agency that handled gestational carriers.

Scenario #2: When Lisa was pregnant with Chris,
she almost died because she had diabetes, a severe
form of high blood pressure, a preclampsia. As a
result, she had suffered an uncontrollable hemor-
rage and had to have a hysterectomy. She and her
husband, David, want Chris to have a brother or sister. They asked Lisa's favorite cousin, Laura, if
she'd carry a baby for them. She said yes.

In both cases, the infertile couple finds a woman
who will donate the use of her uterus to carry their

child. In Carol and Bob's case, they went through an agency. David and Lisa chose to ask a relative.

What to Expect: In this third-party option, IVF is performed using the infertile couple's eggs and sperm. Embryos are transferred to the gestational carrier who has been given hormones to prepare her uterus for embryo implantation. Extra embryos can be frozen for future attempts.

The Pros:

- The child has both the male and female partner's genetic makeup.

- You know something about the gestational carrier's medical history.

- You get to follow the gestational carrier's progress throughout the pregnancy.

- If you use a relative or close friend, you and she may forge an even stronger bond than before.

- You can freeze extra embryos that aren't transferred during IVF.

The Cons:

- You must have good legal counsel to handle the technicalities involved.

- This route is expensive because an IVF procedure is involved and you must pay the gestational carrier's medical expenses.

- The IVF procedure and embryo transfer must be synchronized. The female partner must go through ovulation induction for the IVF procedure. And, the gestational carrier must receive hormones to prepare her uterus for embryo transfer.

- Unless the gestational carrier has had children before, you don't know if she has a fully functioning uterus.

Unofficially...
The first gestational surrogacy procedure was reported in 1985 in the *New England Journal of Medicine*. In this case, the woman's uterus had been removed but her ovaries were intact.

Donor egg/gestational carrier

When the female partner cannot contribute eggs or
use of her uterus, the use of a gestational carrier
may be combined with the use of egg donation. This
is an offshoot of traditional surrogacy and a pairing
of two third-party reproduction methods.

Scenario #1: John and Mary are very anxious to
start a family, especially since Mary had just successfully been treated for uterine cancer. Unfortunately
the treatment involved removing ovaries along with
her uterus. Mary's best friend, Gerry, offers to carry
the child for them as a gestational carrier. But
because she's forty-two, everyone agrees it would be
too risky to use her eggs. They decide to use an
anonymous donor, since they all feel that would be
less complicated than involving another friend.

Scenario #2: Paul and Karen are in their mid-
thirties and had been trying to have a baby for five
years. Karen's had three miscarriages, all occurring
during her second trimester. They don't want to risk
another miscarriage and aren't sure if there's a
genetic component to her miscarriage. Her doctor
suggests using a gestational carrier. They'd like their
child to be as closely related to them as possible, so
they decide to use eggs donated by her sister, Ellen.
Because Ellen doesn't wish to go through a
pregnancy and childbirth—she has a set of twin
toddlers—they go to a surrogacy center and find a
gestational carrier.

Instead of Gerry being inseminated with the
John's sperm and carrying the fetus to term, eggs
from anonymous donor, Ann, are used. In Paul and
Karen's case, they chose a family member as donor,
but still turn to an agency for their gestational carrier. In either case, this option involves four people:

The infertile couple, the woman who donates the eggs, and the woman who carries the fetus.

What to Expect. The donor has to take fertility drugs and the gestational carrier must take hormones to prepare her uterus to accept an embryo transfer, a procedure that is timed to coincide with the availability of the donor's eggs.

The Pros:

- The child has the male partner's genes.

- You can monitor the gestational carrier's medical progress.

The Cons:

- This is expensive because an IVF procedure is involved, you must find and pay the egg donor (if anonymous), as well as for the gestational carrier's medical and legal expenses.

- Because four people are involved, chances of medical and legal complications increase considerably.

Sperm donation, egg donation, gestational carrier

If neither you nor your partner has eggs or sperm to use, and the female partner doesn't have a functioning uterus, either, there are in fact two possible solutions. One is to use donated sperm to fertilize donated eggs via IVF, then transfer the embryos to a gestational carrier. The other solution is one that's been used for centuries: adoption. (See Chapter 9 for more information on the adoption option.)

Scenario #1: Bill and Jean are in their early thirties. Bill is a paraplegic and Jean had had a total hysterectomy several years ago. They don't want to adopt because they want to have some input on the creation of their child. Neither electroejaculation stimulation nor sperm retrieval had yielded viable sperm. They carefully chose an anonymous sperm donor. Jean's sister was willing to be the gestational carrier but she had experienced infertility problems that had been overcome using donor eggs. They found an anonymous egg donor.

Scenario #2: Andrew and Sandy have tried to conceive for ten years. They've exhausted all their options—including IVF, GIFT, and ISCI, and even acupuncture and herbal medicine. Andrew's last sperm count indicated he was virtually sterile, and Sandy, who's in her late forties and diabetic, was told by her doctor that it would be too risky for her to become pregnant. They didn't want to adopt because they were still determined to have a genetic connection to their child. Andrew's brother offered to donate his sperm and Sandy's cousin said she would donate her eggs, but didn't want to go through a pregnancy. A local agency found a gestational carrier for them.

The Pros:

- You can pick each donor involved, including the sperm and egg donors and the gestational carrier.

- Having one or more of the donors known to you provides an added bond to the experience.

The Cons:

- The child would not have any genetic link to you and your partner.

- It's expensive because an IVF procedure is needed.

- It's also expensive because you must arrange for two types of donation, sperm and eggs, as well as for the services and care of the gestational carrier.

■ With the use of any type of known donor third-party reproduction method, the risk of legal complications is increased.

As you can see many of these later options (embryo donation and sperm donation, egg donation, and/or a gestational carrier) seem very much genetically related to adoption—an option that many couples ultimately choose.

Just the facts

■ Egg donations are eliminating many of the reasons to use traditional surrogates.

■ ICSI is eliminating many of the reasons to use sperm donation.

■ Egg donations require coordination of retrieval and IVF procedures.

■ A gestational carrier must take drugs to prepare her uterus for embryo implantation.

■ Agencies specializing in third-party reproduction can help find a suitable donor and take care of legal paperwork.

GET THE SCOOP ON...
High tech innovations ▪ Cryosurgery and
cloning ▪ Acupuncture ▪ Vitamin therapy
and herbal medicine ▪ Homeopathy ▪ Stress
reduction therapy

Back to the Future

T remendous strides have been made in the last two decades in the diagnosis and treatment of infertility. The introduction of assisted reproductive technologies (ARTs) in the early 1980s—perhaps the most dramatic example—has allowed tens of thousands of infertile couples to fulfill their dreams of having children of their own. The first ART procedure, *in vitro fertilization (IVF)*, and its related techniques have helped mainly women, particularly those with severe tubal disease. Now, with the advent of the first micromanipulation technique, *intracytoplasmic sperm insemination (ISCI)*, men who were once considered sterile can now father children, as well.

But there are many hurdles left to overcome to help more infertile couples. This is especially important in light of the National Center for Health Statistics projections that a staggering 7.7 million couples (1.5 million more American couples than in 1995) could be infertile by the year 2025!

Chapter 11

Improving ART success

Although thousands of babies have been born from ART procedures, success rates, while constantly improving, still range from about 20 to 50 percent, depending on the technique and severity of the couple's problem. Researchers are now learning more about why some couples undergoing ART procedures never produce a fertilized egg, have an embryo implant, or maintain an on-going pregnancy.

In addition, doctors are trying to grapple with one of the more troubling aspects of ART: the increased risk of multiple births, particularly triplets, from IVF and related procedures. ASRM guidelines recommend that only three embryos be transferred in young women with good-quality embryos (more, depending on age, embryo quality, and procedure). Some other countries have similar or even more restrictive guidelines and regulations. The reason: The clinical and economic toll that multiple births place on the mother, child, and society.

Researchers and clinicians are exploring better ways to evaluate embryos before they're transferred. This would allow doctors to pick for transfer the one, two, or three embryos with the best chance of producing an on-going pregnancy. It would also dramatically reduce the chance of triplet or quadruplet births because fewer embryos would be needed.

Better embryo evaluation would have other benefits, too. If more first-IVF attempts were successful, fewer embryos would need to be frozen. Right now, specialists fear an overpopulation of cryopreserved embryos with no clear futures. Also, freezing better-quality embryos might mean that later frozen embryo transfer attempts might be more successful.

What fertility specialists learn about embryos may also help the thousands of couples who suffer from spontaneous miscarriages. It's estimated that about 60 percent of spontaneous miscarriages are caused by chromosomal abnormalities in the embryos.

On the horizon

Here is a closer look at some of the promising new reproductive techniques being investigated:

■ **Micromanipulation of eggs.** Researchers and clinicians are now applying some of the same techniques used in intracytoplasmic sperm insemination (ICSI), in which they work on a single sperm, to reconstruct a single human egg. By taking the best components of a donor egg of a younger woman, they are hoping to help older women, and women whose embryos don't seem to develop well, achieve pregnancies. The two types of egg micromanipulation being studied now are:

1. *Oocyte nuclear transfer.* Using very delicate instruments, researchers are removing the gene-packed nucleus of an infertile woman's egg and putting it into a donor egg that has had its nucleus removed. This very experimental technique might one day help older women for whom egg donation is the only viable option. Using a donor's cytoplasm—the portion of the egg surrounding the nucleus that sort of energizes the egg—may be all that's needed to "rejuvenate" the infertile older woman's eggs into fertilizing and developing normally. So far, these experimental reconstructed human eggs seem to start to develop

Unofficially...
A 1996 study of the cost of a successful birth among singletons and twins in one ART practice was about $40,000. In contrast, the cost for triplet and quadruplet pregnancies was approximately $340,000! The major economic burden was due to neonatal intensive care unit charges and ongoing care for infants born under 30 weeks gestation.

normally. Some early success with this technique has been reported. Oocyte nuclear transfer might help women for whom egg donation has been an option, as well as women who have certain types of genetic diseases linked to mitochondria in their cytoplasm. Again, back to biology class: Cytoplasm in our cells contains mitochondria and has it's own set of functioning DNA. Replacing the mitochondria-containing cytoplasm may get rid of the risk of passing on a genetic disorder.

2. *Cytoplasmic transfer.* Akin—in more ways than one—to oocyte nuclear transfer, cytoplasmic transfer works in the opposite direction. In this procedure, a small amount of normal cytoplasm is extracted from a donor egg and injected into an egg of an infertile older woman. Here, again, the donor cytoplasm may give the egg all the boost it needs to produce a pregnancy. So far, this technique has produced only one or two known pregnancies and births.

Here's something else researchers—and maybe you—might consider one day. Because doctors are likely to have extra unused donor eggs when they try a cytoplasmic transfer, they might take some of these unused donor eggs and do an IVF procedure and freeze any developing embryos. If the cytoplasmic transfer doesn't work, the frozen embryos from the donor eggs would be available for the couple to use at a later time. This would be a regular donor egg IVF procedure.

Watch Out!
Oocyte nuclear and cytoplasmic transfers will give a new twist to the third-party reproduction options. With them, a child might actually have two genetic mothers —you and the donor who also supplies part of her eggs!

■ **Preimplantation genetic diagnosis (PGD).** PGD, a recently developed technique, which involves taking a single cell from a newly developing embryo and analyzing its genetic makeup, is offering the promise to help both fertile and infertile couples in have healthy babies. Here are just a few:

1. *Finding chromosomal and genetic disorders early.* Researchers and clinicians are using PGD to test early embryos for various genetic disorders prior to their transfer. Right now, if there's a risk of passing on an hereditary disease, women must undergo an amniocentesis or *chorion villus* sampling in the early months of pregnancy. If the results show the child is in danger of inheriting the disease or genes for the disease, the option is elective abortion—a physically and psychologically traumatizing event. With PGD, the results are known even before an embryo is transferred and a pregnancy occurs. Researchers are hoping that PDG can be used to detect a variety of genetic disorders, such as Duchenne muscular dystrophy, hemophilia, cystic fibrosis, and Tay-Sachs.

2. *Picking good-quality embryos.* Doctors know that one reason some embryos don't implant is that they contain a type of chromosomal abnormality, called *chromosome aneuploidy* or extra chromosome. In fact, some studies have shown that about half the embryos from what doctors call "difficult IVF patients" may have this genetic defect. PGD can be used to detect this

Unofficially...
Nearly a decade ago, researchers reported the first human pregnancies using PGD. In those cases, they were able to determine if the embryo was male or female. A couple of years later, they used PGD to test for cystic fibrosis.

chromosomal abnormality prior to embryo transfer. This would spare an infertile couple repeated unsuccessful treatment cycles because embryos with these defects could be identified and not transferred. Only those without identified defects would be.

3. *Fluorescent in situ hybridization (FISH).* Another highly specialized PGD technique under study, called FISH, uses synthetic DNA segments that have special fluorescent markers attached to them. If the FISH probe tags a genetic target in a chromosome under study, these segments bind ("hybidize") to it and light up. The bright color can signal a chromosomal abnormality, such as extra chromosomes or other genetic abnormalities. A number of genetic diseases, including Tay-Sachs disease, Huntington's disease, Duschenne dystrophy, and cystic fibrosis, have been tested using FISH analysis.

■ **Blastocyst culture of embryos.** Researchers and clinicians are trying to imitate nature's own timing. By delaying transfer until an embryo is a little more developed, they hope to increase the chances of implantation. In IVF, embryos are typically transferred about two or three days after fertilization, when they are in the two- to eight-cell, stage.

Researchers are looking into whether culturing embryos longer before transferring them into the uterus would improve implantation rates. They reason: During natural conception embryos don't implant until about five days after fertilization. At that point they're at the *blastocyst* or greater than eight-cell stage. Culturing embryos longer might also give doctors a longer time to see if the embryos are developing normally and then transfer only the apparently normal ones. This might allow fewer embryos to be transferred to achieve a successful pregnancy and birth, increasing the chance of success and reducing the risk of multiple births.

▪ **In vitro maturation of human eggs.** Researchers are working on ways to help immature eggs mature in the lab. This would reduce the heavy reliance on fertility drugs to boost the number of mature eggs available for retrieval. In essence, the drugs would be given to the eggs rather than the whole person. It would be also be a boon to women who don't seem to respond to fertility drugs, those at high risk of ovarian hyperstimulation, and those who have polycystic ovarian disease.

▪ **Biochemical assisted hatching.** As you saw in Chapter 8, assisted hatching is being used to help improve implantation rates following IVF in older woman. In assisted hatching, chemicals are used to thin or dissect a small area of the outer covering of a human egg, making it easier for the egg to attach to the uterine lining. Doctors are finding that boosting the culture medium in which embryos are grown with chemicals called *proteases* helps improve hatching and pregnancy rates even more.

Unofficially...
Researchers speculate that combining new, improved cryopreservation techniques with in vitro egg maturation may allow women diagnosed with cancer to put their eggs in deep freeze for future use.

▪ **Cryopreservation.** Doctors know that freezing can damage delicate cells. Cells have water in them and when frozen they expand and ice crystals form, which can permanently damage microscopic cellular structures. Cryopreservation uses special fluids, called cryoprotectants, that act very much like car anti-freeze to prevent expansion and crystal formation. Unfortunately, this type of cryoperservation works for some tissues, like sperm and embryos, and not for others, like eggs.

Researchers are experimenting with new coolants and fast cooling times. The new coolants cause the liquids inside the cell to vitrify, that is, form glass rather than freeze and form ice crystals. It's the ice crystals that harm the cells. So far, investigators have been quite successful with mouse eggs and embryos; less so with human ones. It's hoped that better freezing methods would improve pregnancy rates using frozen embryos. Right now, frozen embryos don't do as well as fresh ones, partly because freezing subtly damages the embryo cells.

Better freezing techniques would also allow eggs to be frozen more successfully. So far, there have only been isolated reports of births from frozen eggs. Unfertilized frozen eggs seem very susceptible to damage during freezing and thawing process. Even subtle, undetectable damage may affect embryo development and pregnancy.

Egg donation is providing women who are not producing eggs, as well as older and menopausal women, with the chance to become pregnant. Freezing eggs would allow women who are at risk of loosing ovarian functioning because of drug treatment, radiotherapy, or age to freeze their eggs for later use.

A more likely cryopreservation success may be the freezing of ovarian tissue. Women under chemo- or radiotherapy would then have the option to freeze ovarian tissue. At a later time, the eggs can be retrieved and matured in the lab and used in IVF procedures that would allow these women to have children. This is highly investigative part of ongoing research around the world.

Cloning, cloning, cloning

As you can see, these research efforts may offer hope to thousands of infertile couples, but they also raise important ethical and moral concerns. Perhaps the most controversial of all the techniques is cloning.

Cloning, while intriguing to some, has terrified many. Fear abounds that cloning could be used for ill rather than good. Certainly, the popular Ira Levin book, *The Boys From Brazil*, in which little Hitlers were cloned, reinforced this fear. The only thing that reassured many was that cloning was impossible—or at least not likely to become possible for decades to come.

Much to the dismay of many, however, Scottish researchers were able to clone a sheep—which they named Dolly—in 1998. What makes Dolly and her fellow sheep clones Holly, Molly, and Olly unique is that they were cloned from an adult cell. Dolly is genetically identical to her one parent.

It's pretty easy to make a genetic copy of an animal or even a human being from a fertilized egg. Nature does it often—a fertilized egg splits in two and you have genetically identical twins. If a

Watch Out!
Another futuristic use for cryopreservation might be to freeze eggs from aborted fetuses. The ovaries of these fetuses might be rich with potentially useable eggs. This would mean that a woman could have a child who's actually her grandchild—but that "grandchild" actually had no birth mother.

blastomere were separated deliberately in the lab it might be called "assisted twinning."

The cloning upon which science fiction stories are based—and which Dolly represents—involves making a genetically identical copy from an adult cell. Each cell in our body contains all the genetic information that makes us who we are. We know that a cell from our liver contains the genes that makes us have black hair or blue eyes. Pretty soon after conception our cells begin to *differentiate* or become and continue to become a specific type of cell. Once a cell becomes differentiated to be a brain cell, for example, it doesn't become a liver cell.

But, could you get a cell to "forget" becoming a particular type of cell and start becoming a whole new organism again—just like it did when it was first fertilized and began to divide? In layman's terms, here's what Dolly's lab "parents" did:

1. They took a sheep egg cell and removed its nucleus.

2. They took cells from a sheep (the Scottish researchers used cells from a sheep's udder) and cultured them in the lab.

3. They managed to starve the cells just enough to trick them into a sort of hybernating state. It wasn't enough to kill the cells, but it was enough to stop them from "differentiating" or continuing to grow into udder cells.

4. They put the udder cell under the outer cell membrane of the hollowed-out egg cell. Then they zapped them with an electrical charge.

5. The jolt fused the two cells together and the nucleus of the udder cells became the nucleus of the egg and the new cell began to act like a fertilized egg.

6. This egg was transferred and then implanted—like regular run of the mill IVF—into a sheep gestational carrier.

7. Dolly was born.

Complementary and alternative medicine

Some of the newest approaches to infertility treatments have their roots in some of the oldest forms of medicine—ancient Eastern cultures dating back thousands of years. These non-traditional medical treatmentss have been commonly referred to as *alternative medicine.* *Integrative medicine* is another term for this approach, and it is the term primarily used by medical professionals. However, both traditional and non-traditional practitioners now generally refer to these treatments as *complementary and alternative medicine,* or CAM.

Whatever it's called, CAM is becoming recognized as a legitimate component in the management of many conditions, including infertility. Researchers and doctors have finally realized that alternative medicine is more than just aphrodisiacs and fertility statues. They are catching up with consumers in their acknowledgment of the potential benefits of CAM for many conditions. Several medical publications, including the prestigious *Journal of the American Medical Association (JAMA),* have recently called for manuscripts on CAM. JAMA's editorial advisory board has selected alternative medicine as one of the top three subjects for future journal issues.

A staggering number of Americans, an estimated 83 million people or 40 percent of adults in this country, turn to CAM for various conditions. They

"

Recent develop-
ments indicate
changing atti-
tudes toward
these unconven-
tional therapies,
and demonstrate
increasing recog-
nition of the
need to critically
investigate the
safety and
efficacy of com-
plementary and
alternative medi-
cine practices
and to determine
how some of
these therapies
could be
integrated into
clinical practice
to improve
patient care.
—*Journal of the
American Medical
Association,*
December 19,
1997

"

are spending over $27 million on such treatments as acupuncture, chiropractics, homeopathy, or other therapies that fall under the CAM umbrella. And one in three people in the U.S. use non-traditional medical alternatives on a regular basis. In fact, in 1990, more visits were made to CAM providers than primary care physicians!

Spawned by thousands of anecdotal reports and a growing body of legitimate study results—and a Congressional mandate—the National Institutes of Health (NIH) established the U.S. Office of Alternative Medicine in 1992 to help formalize research on the use, safety, and effectiveness of a broad range of nontraditional therapies. Now called the *National Center for Complementary and Alternative Medicine (NCCAM)*, it has an annual budget of more than $40 million. NCCAM currently funds CAM research at 10 research centers across the country.

Over 300 complementary and alternative medicine therapies have been documented in the U.S., which NCCAM groups under the seven major categories listed below:

- Mind-body interventions. These include stress management, hypnosis, imagery, tai chi, qi dong, and yoga.

- Alternative systems of medical practice. These include acupuncture, naturopathic medicine, Native American practices, traditional Oriental medicine, and past life therapy.

- Manual healing methods. This category includes acupressure, chiropractics, massage therapy, reflexology, and therapeutic touch.

- Pharmacologic and biologic treatments. Chelation therapy and antioxidising treatments fall under this category.

- Bioelectromagnetic applications. This category include artificial lighting, electrostimulation, and electroacupuncture.

- Herbal medicine. Common medicinal herbs include echinacea, ginger rhizomes, ginkgo biloba extract, ginseng root and St. John's Wort.

- Diet and nutrition. Lifestyle changes, macrobiotics, megavitamins, and nutritional supplements are all under this category.

According to a 1993 article in the *New England Journal of Medicine*, the most commonly used alternative medical treatments in this country are biofeedback, exercise, prayer, relaxation techniques, and yoga.

CAM and infertility

While there are no statistics on how many infertile men and women seek CAM treatments, if the national average holds true, at least one third do. The American Society for Reproductive Medicine (ASRM) has published articles in the journal *Fertility and Sterility* on CAM practices, especially stress reduction, and RESOLVE has a fact sheet on naturopathic medicine and acupuncture. Besides these CAMs, others that are popular among people with fertility problems are relaxation techniques, yoga, support groups, herbal medicine and homeopathy.

Below we will briefly describe some of those CAMs that have been, at least to some extent, evaluated or reported on in medical journals with regard to the treatment of infertility problems. We want to stress that the following is for informational purposes only. We are not recommending any of these methods. If you are considering trying any of them be sure to discuss it with your physician first.

Timesaver
Using the Internet is an easily accessible, quick source of information about CAMs. You might want to start with NIH's NCCAM at http://altmed. od.nih.gov. They also have links to many other CAM Internet sites.

Unofficially...
The New Scientist Magazine reported that a scientist in Liverpool, England, found that men with long ring fingers and symmetrical hands had higher levels of testosterone and produced more sperm than men with asymmetrical hands and short ring fingers. He also discovered that women had higher levels of estrogen if their first fingers were longer than their third fingers.

Bright Idea
If you're inter-
ested in trying
acupuncture, be
sure to ask the
acupuncturist to
use disposable
needles. This will
reduce the risk
of infection.

Acupuncture

Acupuncture is an ancient Chinese medical system that has been practiced for over 3,000 years in the East. Chinese medicine believes that disease disrupts the flow of healthy energy, called Qi and pronounced "chee." Acupuncture is used to correct the imbalance of energy flow by stimulating acupuncture points on the body with very thin needles, heat (moxibustion), massage, electrical stimulation, and occasionally herbs.

Acupuncture became popular in the U.S. in the early 1970's among both consumers and physicians. Today, there are approximately 10,000 practicing acupuncturists in this country alone, and 4,000 of them are physicians. Indeed, the number of acupuncturists practicing in the U.S. is expected to double by the year 2000. And, according to the FDA, approximately one million Americans spend about $500 million on acupuncture each year.

"
Ideally, CAM
practices have
the potential for
filling in and
supplying needs
where conven-
tional medicine
may not be
completely
satisfactory.
—Wayne B.
Jonas, MD,
Director, NIH's
OAM, in an
interview pub-
lished in the
specialty medical
magazine,
*Contemporary
OB/GYN*,
February, 1998.
"

While acupuncture is most often thought of as a method of pain relief, it has many other applications including the treatment of infertility. According to Chinese medicine, infertility can be caused by such conditions as "deficient blood" and "cold womb" and "weak kidney energy," and acupuncture and herbs can successfully treat these conditions. A 1997 review article of CAM therapies published in *Obstetrical and Gynecological Survey* reported one study in which infertile women who had undergone acupuncture were found to be more likely to become pregnant and have fewer miscarriages than a control group. In another study, conducted in Israel and published in 1997 in the *Archives of Andrology*, acupuncture was found to improve sperm motility in subfertile men.

Vitamin therapy

As we all know, vitamins and minerals are essential to maintaining good health. Research is increasingly being conducted on the preventive and curative effects of certain vitamins and minerals. For example, a study on sperm motility in infertile men was conducted in Glasgow, Scotland. The results, which were published in the *British Journal of Urology* in 1998, found that supplements of selenium improved sperm motility in some subfertile men, and, as a result, increased the chances of successful pregnancy in their partners. Selenium is found primarily in whole grains and eggs, and is also available as a supplement. Be careful: Doses greater than 200 mcg can be toxic.

Vitamins and minerals such as Vitamin E, Vitamin C, Vitamin B_6, Vitamin B_{12}, and zinc are purported to enhance fertility in both men and women. Zinc and Vitamin B_6 have been reported to be especially useful for male infertility and impotence. Antioxidants in general are believed to protect sperm from toxic damage.

Certain foods, especially soy products, flax seeds, and yams contain natural estrogens and have been used to treat menopause. They may also prove to be a useful adjunct to the treatment of infertility.

Keep in mind, however, that this list is incomplete: The results of studies on many other vitamins and minerals are just starting to come in, and not all vitamins and minerals have been tested. So no claims of efficacy can be made or implied. And remember, just because something is "natural," don't assume it's safe.

Herbal medicine

Herbs and plant derivatives have been the basis for medical treatments for thousands of years.

Watch Out!
If you *do* become pregnant, do not take any drug, vitamin, herb or other CAM without first consulting your obstetrician. Even if a label says the product can be taken during pregnancy, or can be used to prevent miscarriages, it may not be safe for you. Trust your doctor, not the label.

According to the Bible, Rachael, who poignantly lamented, "Give me children or else I die!" finally conceived after eating mandrakes, a root that is shaped like a man.

About half the medications used in Western medicine are plant-based. These include many of our most accepted, effective, and popular drugs such as aspirins, digitalis, cascara, and taxol, a new drug currently being used to treat breast and ovarian cancer. These drugs are tried and true and have been through rigorous testing in animals and humans. Most of the herbs used by herbalists, however, have not yet gone through the necessary research trials to prove them safe and effective. But this is rapidly changing, with government funds being poured into evaluating the safety and effectiveness of these herbal remedies. Time—and testing—will tell.

The following are just a sampling of some of the herbal preparations purported, but not necessarily proven, to have helped some infertile men and women:

- *Ho Shou Wu,* a Chinese herb, is used to treat female infertility and, in fact, has been demonstrated to be effective in animal studies.

- *Vitex agnus catus* has been shown to affect the pituitary gland's secretion of progesterone and may help in correcting for imbalances in progesterone and estrogen levels.

- *Dong quai,* another Chinese herb, is known as the Queen of Female Herbs, and said to balance and nourish the female reproductive system.

- *False Unicorn Root* has one of the best reputations among herbalists for enhancing fertility, and is often used to treat ovarian dysfunction.

- *Chamaelirium luteum* is used treat impotency and female infertility, as well as prevent miscarriages.

- *Alertris farinosa* (True Unicorn Root) is another herb that has been said to help prevent miscarriages. It also supposedly can help cure impotence, as does Yohimbine Bark.

Homeopathy

Homeopathy was developed 200 years ago by Samuel Hahneman, a German physician and chemist. Homeopathy is form of medicine that uses highly diluted doses of medicine usually derived from herbs, plants, and minerals to stimulate the body's own defense mechanisms to cure various disorders.

Most homeopaths in the U.S. are medical doctors who attend four years of regular medical school and then specialize in homeopathic medicine. Homeopathy is also popular with other licensed medical professionals, especially naturopaths, acupuncturists, chiropractors, physicians, nurses, dentists, and veterinarians. There are three recognized, accredited schools of homeopathy that can train these health professionals in a three or four year programs. However, not all homeopathic training programs require that the student have prior medical training. Several professional organizations certify or license homeopaths.

Homeopathy claims to be useful in the treatment of endometriosis, and in helping to shrink both cysts and fibroids, although fibroids are said to take longer to treat. Homeopathic treatment for these conditions should be done through a homeopathic physician. Self-treatment should be avoided.

Moneysaver
Check ahead of time to see if your insurance policy covers CAM visits. Increasing numbers of insurance companies are now paying for visit to CAM practitioners such as acupuncturists, homeopaths, naturopaths and chiropractors.

Bright Idea
If you're plan-
ning to take an
herbal prepara-
tion, rather than
taking a full
dosage right
away, take a
small amount a
day for a few
days and monitor
yourself for aller-
gic reactions or
other side
effects. If you
have them, don't
take that herb.
Always check
with your doctor
before taking
any herbal
preparation.

Stress reduction

Since the 1960's when Harvard researchers found
that relaxation techniques could lower blood pressure, the mind-body connection has been looked
into with growing acceptance.

In a 1998 study reported in ASRM's *Fertility and
Sterility*, Belgian researchers found that women who
were depressed but had good coping skills got pregnant through IVF more often than depressed
women undergoing IVF who didn't have such skills.
It's difficult, however, to evaluate whether being
depressed just makes you less likely to follow treatment instructions or whether depression can upset
hormone balance.

Reporting at the 1998 meeting of the ASRM, a
Massachusetts psychologist reported that group
therapy seemed to help improve the chance of pregnancy among a group of infertile women. Group
therapy and support groups provide invaluable
information, motivate members to make positive
decisions about their treatment, and steer members
toward the best doctors and most effective treatments. All of these factors, rather than the therapy
per se, are likely to result in higher pregnancy rates.

As we have pointed out in many places in this
book, stress can be the result of infertility, but there
is very little evidence that it is a significant factor in
infertility. You can't just relax and get pregnant. But
relaxing certainly doesn't hurt—on the contrary, it
can help keep you fit to meet the physical and emotional challenges of infertility diagnosis and treatment. And relaxing may just help you do the things
necessary to increase your chances of conceiving.
Relieving stress can increase your desire to have
and/or ability to have intercourse. It can also make
it easier for you to undergo unpleasant and invasive

tests and treatments such as hysterosalpinograms and IVF. When people are under less stress, they are more likely to remember to take their medication at the right time, and have sex at the right time.

Stress reduction and relaxation techniques can also help you in your everyday lives, going through a pregnancy or adoption, and dealing with a newborn, and later, toddlers and teenagers. And there certainly are no counter indications for or negative side effects from stress reduction. It can be used as an adjunct to any medical treatment, no matter what your diagnosis is.

Naturopathic medicine

If you're interested in pursing a CAM treatment for infertility but are not certain as to which one would be best, you may want to consider seeing a naturopathic doctor (N.D.) Naturopathic medicine, while having its roots in ancient medicine, was developed in the U.S. about 100 years ago by Benjamin Lust. Naturopathic medicine focuses on prevention and treating the whole person through the healing power of nature. N.D.s use a wide variety of natural treatments including homeopathy, nutritional and vitamin therapy, acupuncture, Ayurvedic (Indian) medicine, native American medicine, herbal medicine, and stress management.

There are over 1,000 licensed naturopathic physicians in this country. Only two schools in this country, however, are presently accredited, Bastyr University of Natural Health Sciences in Seattle, Washington, and National College of Naturopathic Medicine in Portland, Oregon. Bastyr, in fact, is one of the research sites funded by NIH's Office of Alternative Medicine. N.D.s from accredited schools undergo four years of medical studies similar to what standard medical schools require. Just as you

Watch Out!
Some individuals use the initials N.D. after their names after only completing a mail-order course. They lack the necessary training to effectively and safely treat many conditions, and cannot obtain licenses in those states that license naturopaths.

check out a doctor's credentials, make sure you check out an N.D.'s credentials.

About 70 insurance companies in the U.S. cover treatment by licensed naturopaths. At present, coverage for naturopathic medicine is mandatory in two states, Washington and Connecticut.

Going the alternative route

If you're considering trying one of the above or some other CAM therapies, here are a few things to keep in mind:

- Before starting any CAM therapy, be sure to tell your doctor. He or she must know what you're considering to insure that it won't interfere with other aspects of your current or planned fertility treatment. Some herbal products or megadoses of combination nutritional supplements can be harmful, or they might interfere with the medicines your fertility doctor is prescribing. Other practices, like acupuncture, when properly done, probably won't have any negative effect on traditional treatments. So while your doctor may be skeptical, he or she shouldn't dismiss your pursing CAM unless it will interfere with your fertility treatment, or be detrimental to you or a developing fetus.

- Find a CAM provider the same way you would any other medical provider—by taking the time to check out all your options and caregivers. Start by rereading Chapter 3 on finding the right doctor.

- If possible, choose a *licensed* CAM provider. Many practitioners of nontraditional medicine must be licensed and belong to professional organizations that set practice standards.

For example, every state requires chiropractors to be licensed, and most states require acupuncturists to be licensed as well. Acupuncturists who are medical doctors are automatically licensed. Naturopathic practitioners and massage therapists are also required to be licensed in some states.

- Find out where the practitioner trained and whether or not he or she completed the training program. Also find out what, if any, professional organizations she or he belongs to.

- Try to get information about the training institute or program—such as whether or not it's accredited—in order to ascertain it's legitimacy.

- Interview the practitioner. Ask: "Do you have a working relationship with traditional doctors in your area?" "Are you affiliated with a hospital?" "What experience do you have in working with infertility patients?"

- Talk to some of the practitioner's or clinic's patients. While testimonials should be taken with a grain of salt, they do give some indication as to the effectiveness of a practitioner, from at least the patient's perspective.

- Try only one CAM at a time. More than one approach can be counterproductive.

- If a technique doesn't work in a few months, don't continue it. Of course, a CAM therapy such as yoga, which helps you in general, doesn't need to be abandoned. Regardless of its direct effectiveness on resolving your fertility problems, keeping your mind and body healthy and relaxed is probably the best thing you can do for yourself.

Unofficially...
Be careful about generalizing from testimonials and anecdotal stories of success of any particular alternative treatment. While interesting, anecdotal evidence cannot be used to prove that a treatment is successful or not. Only scientifically controlled studies that include many subjects can definitively prove the effectiveness of a treatment.

Just the facts

- Complementary and alternative medicines have achieved serious medical attention, and are becoming recognized as a legitimate component of the treatment of infertility.

- New genetic testing methods are being used to detect disorders *before* an embryo is transfered.

- Better freezing techniques may prove less damaging to embryos than methods presently in use.

- Acupunctures, and vitamin and herbal therapy appear to show some promise in the treatment of male and female infertility.

- Stress reduction can help you survive the emotional and physical pain of infertility treatment, as well as increase your chances of conception by helping you make the right decisions.

- Your fertility doctor should be consulted before you begin any CAM therapy, to avoid the possibility of negative effects of the CAM treatment on your other treatment options.

The Social, Emotional,
and Financial
Side of Infertility

PART VI

GET THE SCOOP ON...
Surviving scheduled sex ▪ Avoiding marital
conflicts ▪ Strengthening your marriage

The Infertile Marriage

No marital relationship is left unscathed by infertility—it's a major life crisis that can wreak havoc upon the best of marriages. But it doesn't have to. In this chapter, we'll look at some of the common marital problems infertile couples face, some solutions to those problems, and some ways to forge a stronger marriage from the adversity that infertility issues often cause.

...And doctor makes three

When you first decided to have children, it may have crossed your mind that a baby might come between you and your partner at times—especially in the bedroom. It probably never occurred to you, however, that it would be your quest for a baby, not the baby him- or herself, that would disrupt your sex life. And it probably never crossed your mind that your doctor would become involved in the most intimate areas of your life, telling you when to have sex, how often to have sex, and sometimes even *how* to have sex.

Chapter 12

When sex—normally a private, personal matter—becomes part of medical diagnosis and treatment, the results can be disastrous for the couple. Prior to infertility, most infertile couples have normal, happy sex lives. Infertility can put an end to all that, at least temporarily.

The doctor's involvement in the couple's sex life usually starts when the doctor asks the man to produce a sperm sample by masturbation for semen analysis. On the surface, this request seems innocuous enough. But many men are embarrassed, annoyed, and even humiliated by this apparently simple, but critical, request. Their partners, on the other hand, tend not to have much sympathy for their feelings. After all, they themselves have to go through invasive, possibly painful diagnostic procedures, while all the men have to do is masturbate, something that is actually pleasurable. Said one woman, "What's the big deal, jerking off into a jar? But he resents showing up late to work because of it. He says that it make him feel more tense at work, and that he feels tense enough already."

The reality is that most men do resent being told by their doctors that they have to masturbate. In fact, this is probably the first time that they've been ordered to do something that many as youngsters had been taught was "wrong." But throughout infertility treatments, doctors will need to periodically ask for sperm samples for re-evaluation. Some men get used to it; others get increasingly annoyed.

Unless a donor is being used, the husband also has to produce sperm for medical procedures such as artificial insemination and in vitro fertilization. If he refuses to cooperate, he can ruin the couple's chance of a pregnancy for that entire month. And every month counts, especially for older women. It's understandable, then, that wives often become furious when their husbands balk at producing semen.

Adding insult to injury

Men find it especially humiliating when a female receptionist or nurse requests a sperm sample. Said one man, "When the nurse handed me the jar, everyone in the waiting room knew what I was going in the bathroom to do. I was so embarrassed!" Some men find it very difficult to "perform" and are grateful when the bathrooms are equipped with adult magazines or other incentives.

If your spouse gets upset about or refuses to produce a sperm sample, here are some things you can do to ease the situation:

- Be sympathetic. Tell him you understand how difficult this is for him, and you appreciate his cooperation—and contribution.

- Don't pressure. It will only anger him and make things worse.

- Provide a helping hand. Offer to accompany your husband when he has to produce a sperm sample. He may appreciate the help and it can be fun for both of you.

- Lighten up. Try to see the humor in the situation. Others certainly do. You can start by checking out the following web site that deals with infertility and humor: http://www.inciid.org/humor.html. But keep in mind that your partner may not see any humor in the situation, at least at first.

Unofficially... Many IVF programs have "Masturbatoriums" for the men. These softly lit, comfortable rooms are usually equipped with VCRs, X-rated tapes, and adult magazines.

Things may get worse before they get better

As the infertility workup and treatment progress, your doctor very quickly becomes privy to your love life. While taking your medical history, your doctor will directly ask about your frequency of sexual intercourse, its timing, and even the positions you customarily use. In addition, if your doctor hasn't already done so, he or she may ask the woman to keep a temperature chart for three months (see Chapter 4). Besides recording your basal temperature, your doctor may also want you to mark the days when you and your partner have sexual intercourse.

Scheduled sex

The dreaded scheduled sex usually starts when the doctor orders a postcoital exam. In retrospect, producing semen upon request and answering questions about your sex life may by this point have begun to seem easy. To do a postcoital exam correctly, your doctor will tell you to have intercourse on certain days around ovulation. As we mentioned in Chapter 4, a postcoital exam requires that the couple have sex the night or morning before the exam.

Your doctor will also probably tell you to have intercourse on certain predetermined days each month, right around the time of ovulation. So much for spontaneity! Your sex life will no longer primarily be dictated by love, affection, or sexual desire, but by your doctor and thermometer. It's no wonder that scheduled sex often leads to marital and sexual problems.

Because of this pressure to perform on demand, it's also not unusual for men to have bouts of impotency and to begin to have trouble achieving or

Watch Out!
Many couples exaggerate the number of times they have intercourse in a given month. It is not a good idea to do this when reporting to your doctor, because it's very important for diagnostic purposes that there be an accurate record of when and how often you have sex.

maintaining an erection. And scheduled sex takes its toll on women as well. Many infertile women find they have difficulty reaching an orgasm, or are totally uninterested in sex for anything except procreation. One woman described her sex life as follows: "I think my husband knows that I'm lying there thinking, just deposit the sperm and leave. Which is all I'm interested in. I'm not interested in sex anymore. I'm interested in conception.... If I could take a little pill in the morning instead of having sex, I would rather do that—that would be wonderful."

Scheduled abstinence

Just when you've come to terms with scheduled sex, you might find yourself confronted with another problem—scheduled abstinence. There are times throughout a treatment cycle when a doctor might tell you not to have sex at certain times. For example, the doctor may feel that abstaining a few days before ovulation can build up your partner's sperm count if it's low.

On top of that, if you do conceive, your doctor may tell you to abstain for last few months because of concerns about possible infection. Telling couples not to have sex can be just as problematic as telling them when to have sex.

A vicious cycle

After going through month after month of infertility, sexual intercourse can start to feel like a futile effort. When conception continually fails to occur, sex is often seen as the culprit, even if the problem is unrelated to intercourse. So sex becomes not only a routine and sometimes difficult chore, but dreaded and unsatisfying, too. As one woman put it,

Bright Idea
If your partner is having sexual problems, you may find it helpful to become more subtle, seductive, and even secretive when you're ovulating. Even if your spouse catches on, you have nothing to lose.

"You're going through the motions of something that time and again has been proven clinically to be unsuccessful. Unless you have absolutely no brains and no sensibilities or sensitivities, you've got to be affected by all that negative reinforcement."

Surviving scheduled sex

66

Scheduled sex made us the best of friends and for a long time very lousy sex partners.
—Wendy, a thirty-eight-year-old nurse

99

Scheduled sex combined with the mood changes caused by both fertility drugs and continued failure to conceive can't help but adversely affect a marriage. Sexual intercourse—a once spontaneous act of love and sexual desire—can become a chore, a duty, a medical prescription often devoid of any feelings of sexuality or even affection. As one woman described her sex life, "There was very little making love. It was mostly making babies."

So it's virtually impossible to have a normal sexual relationship, and therefore a normal marital relationship during infertility treatment.

You might be thinking that things will never be the same again, sexually. But there are things you can do to try to put the spice back into your sex life. Try to do things differently—things that will help you separate sex from conception. Here are a few suggestions that may appeal to you and your partner:

- Concentrate on making love, not babies.
- Experiment with different positions.
- Have oral or other nonprocreative sex when you're not ovulating.
- Have sex when you're not ovulating.
- Have sex in places other than the bedroom.
- Rent X-rated movies.

Fertility fights

Sex is not the only aspect of the marital relationship to suffer from infertility. Couples are likely to fight over any number of issues related to infertility—and sometimes over issues that are not so related. The following woman described how infertility affected her, her husband, and their marriage:

> My husband started getting depressed about the fact that the news was getting worse and worse. He was also starting to see that my patience and psychic energy to continue was being used up. I was starting to consider all the options—everything from continuing trying to never having children. He was very angry that I was no longer so committed to trying to conceive, that there was the possibility of my quitting. He became very hostile to me and criticized everything that I did. My hair was parted in the wrong place. I served too much soup or too little soup. He was constantly criticizing me. I was really aware that he was really angry at me, but I don't think I was aware, at that point, of how angry I was at him. When we finally sat down and talked about it, all those complaints translated into, "You're not dealing with this the way I would do it."

In order to avoid conflict and fights, it's important to respect each other's differing reactions, actions, and emotions. The following are some other helpful hints for maintaining a peaceful marriage:

- Don't blame each other...or yourself.
- Don't hurt each other's feelings.
- Talk it over. Be open with each other about your feelings, concerns, and limits.

Timesaver
If you're having serious sexual problems that you feel may permanently damage your relationship, consult a sex or family therapist immediately. It's better to do it now before things get even worse.

Bright Idea
If you find you can't solve your marital problems, consider joining RESOLVE or another couple's group. Or if you prefer, see a family therapist who has some expertise in treating infertile couples.

- Empathize with each other.
- Be a united team. It's important to keep in mind that the two of you are striving for the same goal—a family.

Whose fault is it anyway?

When couples fight, they commonly blame, insult, and accuse each other of all kinds of things. At some point, you may find yourself blaming your partner for the way he or she deals with infertility—or for being infertile in the first place. This might be especially tempting if your spouse has the primary fertility problem, such as blocked tubes or a low sperm count. But even if you are the one with the primary problem, you may still find reasons to blame your spouse, perhaps for waiting too long to try to conceive, or waiting too long to call an infertility specialist.

Some people feel so convinced that their partners are to blame that they start fantasizing that if they had married someone else, they'd have several children by now. Others even fantasize about having an affair with someone more fertile. Fortunately, most people don't act upon these fantasies. The reality is that you may not be any more likely to conceive with another partner than the one you're with now. One woman described her temptations this way:

> I have thought in my really dark moments that maybe it's just my chemistry with my husband that's not working out. Maybe I should contact an old boyfriend or something. Not for an affair, not for kicks. But just for the right sperm, in my search for this master sperm that can find its way to this very obviously elusive egg.

But blaming your spouse will not get you any closer to a pregnancy, and can only hurt your relationship. Your partner probably feels guilty enough as it is, and doesn't need to be reminded of his or her contribution to your fertility problem.

Both partners, in fact, are likely to have some feelings of guilt and self-blame about their fertility difficulties, regardless of who has the primary medical problem. They may blame themselves for something they did in the past—such as having had an abortion, an affair or numerous sex partners—and feel that infertility is their punishment for their past "crime." They may even offer their spouses a divorce out of guilt over not being able to please them by giving them the one thing they want—a baby.

Blame, whether it's directed toward oneself or one's spouse is counterproductive. It doesn't bring you closer to achieving a pregnancy, and it certainly doesn't help the marriage. Guilt and blame can only lead to depression, anger, and marital tension, when what is really needed is unified action.

Fertility rights...and wrongs

Most of the marital problems infertile couples have are the result of the differences in the way infertility affects each partner. Each is likely to have different emotional reactions and coping styles from those of his or her their partner. For example, one partner may become despondent, pessimistic, and passive. The other may be more optimistic, see infertility as a challenge, and take charge of the situation. One spouse may wish to talk about it endlessly and join a support group while the other prefers to remain silent on the subject and shuns all association with other infertile couples.

Unofficially...
An Orthodox Jewish man can divorce his wife if the couple doesn't conceive, even if the man is sterile.

There is no right or wrong reaction to infertility, as long as your reaction doesn't hurt your spouse or your chances to conceive. Each partner has a right to deal with infertility in a way that helps him or her cope. Each spouse also has to respect and understand his or her partner's emotional reaction and coping methods to avoid conflicts and arguments. But this is easier said than done. Each partner's differing reactions to infertility can't help but cause some friction and fights. Being aware of potential problem areas can help you avoid them, or at least lessen their impact.

While we prefer to avoid sexual stereotyping, many reactions to infertility are, in fact, gender related. For example, most women believe that infertility is both emotionally and physically harder on them than on their spouses, and most men agree. The reality is that men can better distance themselves—both emotionally and physically—from the infertility than can women. Said one woman about her husband's response to infertility, "He's like the stereotype of a man who is able to suppress it all, and goes to work...it just doesn't have the same meaning and terror for him."

Infertility does seem to have a greater personal and biological impact on women than on men. They also have a more difficult time putting infertility out of their minds. This may be because women are ultimately the ones who will or will not become pregnant and give birth. Because of the emotional and physical involvement in their infertility treatment, women tend to think about it, talk about it, and obsess about it more than do men. Most men only think about it when they have to, such as in the doctor's office or when they're actively involved in a diagnostic or treatment procedure. A common result is that men become angry with their partners for making infertility a focal point of their lives, and women get angry with their partners for being uninvolved, unsympathetic, and uncaring. If the husband feels too overwhelmed by his wife's preoccupation with infertility, he may become angry, withdraw, or even belittle her for what he sees as a useless obsession. This has the potential to explode into huge arguments. To avoid these arguments, it's important to understand why infertility is likely to become a major preoccupation, if not an obsession, for most women, but not for men.

Obsessing about infertility

Women tend to obsess about infertility because its diagnosis and treatment quickly become an integral part of their everyday lives. As we have seen in the previous chapters, infertility treatment for women requires frequent doctor's appointments and close monitoring of a woman's menstrual cycle. So even if a woman tries to forget about her infertility, she has constant reminders: Every morning the first thing she does is put a thermometer in her mouth. Every time she goes to the bathroom, she may look for menstrual blood or check the quality of her cervical mucous. Every time she and her husband make love, she wonders if this time it worked, or whether they were wasting time and sperm because she was not ovulating. As one woman described, "It's with me every single day. I wake up with it, I go to sleep with it, and I think about it literally fifty times a day. It is always with me. I dream about it. It's night and day, and day and night, seven days a week ever since this began."

Unlike women, men—even those who are diagnosed as having a fertility problem—do not have these constant reminders of their infertility. Said another woman, "For three years it's been a constant, like my heartbeat."

Withdrawal symptoms

Because of all the attention their wives pay to infertility, many husbands become angry, resentful, and withdrawn emotionally. If the husband has the primary fertility problem, he may also feel guilty that he can't impregnate his wife and might become even more emotionally distant or upset.

When a man retreats emotionally, his partner is likely to feel hurt first, then angry. She might lash out and accuse him of not caring about her and their future family. She'll most likely feel that he's uninvolved and unsupportive and she'll long for both a child *and* her husband. As a result, she may become even more preoccupied with infertility and withdraw from her husband, perpetuating a vicious cycle.

Involving your spouse

One way to help counter this problem is to have your partner more involved in infertility by bringing him with you to the doctor whenever possible. Most women, in fact, prefer to have their partners accompany them to the doctor's office. Although not always necessary for medical reasons, it's reassuring and helpful to have your partner there for emotional support. This is especially true when you have to undergo treatment or tests that are invasive, potentially painful, or anxiety provoking, or when the test or treatment results are crucial in determining the your chances of conceiving.

One woman, herself a doctor, was upset by what she considered her husband's lack of involvement in her medical treatment:

I felt he wasn't as concerned about infertility as I was, that I was doing most of the work. I was the one who had to go to the doctor. I was the one who had to get the injections. I was the one who had to make the appointments, and call the doctor, and get follow-up and get the lab tests, and schlep him there. And I was the one who kept bringing it up for discussion, like when should we think about adoption? Or when should I change doctors? Or should I have the laparoscopy?

The problem is, however, that many men do not see their ongoing presence at doctors' appointments as necessary, much less desirable. While most men are cooperative about going to the doctor when it's absolutely necessary, they resist and then resent it when they don't believe it's essential. This, too, can cause marital tension, as the woman above discovered:

Each time I needed him to come to the doctor with me, I'd have to fight for it. I'd say, "Remember, tomorrow we're going to the doctor." And he'd say, "Oh, I forgot. I have a meeting." And I'd say, "I'd really like you to come with me." And he'd say, "Oh, okay, all right. I'll cancel the meeting"—this whole big martyr schtick.

Talking it over

Throughout this *Unofficial Guide* we've urged you to think about some of the steps you might be taking on your journey through infertility diagnosis and treatment. We've encouraged you to explore the

Moneysaver
One way to save some money and involve your husband in your treatments is to have him give you your hormone shots. And in addition to saving money, playing doctor can be fun!

ramifications of your options and to talk over your views with your partner. We've also pointed out that it's not unusual for your feelings to change as you move through the treatment process. Keeping the lines of communication open, then, is a key to avoiding the myriad marital problems that infertility can cause. Each partner must try to understand and accept the other's feelings, as well as keep the discussions going. You need to talk about infertility: What it means to both of you, what concerns you, and what it's doing to your marriage?

When the woman above and her husband finally sat down to talk about what they were going through, it was a revelation to her. "He said, 'You know, last night when you told me that you'd gotten your period, I felt like you stabbed me. And I realized that even though you accuse me of not being concerned about it, I really am. In fact, I'm so concerned that I can't even deal with it. It's really hard for me.' And we both started crying."

Ironically, the desire to talk about infertility can actually cause tremendous friction in marriages. For most women, talking about infertility helps them cope. In general, women are more comfortable talking about feelings and discussing personal issues than are men. But a wife's need to talk about their infertility can alienate her spouse. It's an unwelcome and seemingly constant reminder of his failure to get her pregnant.

Men also tend to find the topic of infertility boring, while many women find it infinitely interesting. This is similar to the different interests men and women have in discussing pregnancy and childbirth. In fact, infertility can create the same kind of jealousy that a newborn does in many marriages. The husband feels excluded and unneeded when his

> 66
> I knew things were screwed up in our marriage when my husband was giving me shots and the doctor was giving me sperm!
> —Chloe, a thirty-seven-year-old writer.
> 99

previously attentive wife focuses solely on the baby. During infertility treatment, some men feel that their wives' yearning and quest for a baby is interfering in their relationship. The husband may resent the child before he or she is even conceived.

Women frequently want and need to talk about infertility treatments and options with their husbands. This can also cause misunderstandings and conflicts in a marriage, especially if the wife calls her husband at work. Although infertility is probably the last thing a man wants to discuss at the office, his spouse may have to call him to discuss the result of a test, or to schedule an appointment for an insemination, or for comfort after bad news.

Many women complain that their husbands are also reluctant to discuss infertility with friends or relatives, and this too often becomes another area of conflict. Some husbands even forbid their wives to talk about infertility with anyone. Some women cope with infertility by making it the focus of their lives. They don't hesitate to reveal their infertile status to virtually all their acquaintances, and many strangers. Many men, on the other hand, try to ignore or deny their infertility. Said one woman, "My husband found infertility very embarrassing, and I guess he felt emasculated. So he wouldn't talk about it. He would rather have people assume that if we didn't have children, it was because we didn't want children."

Talking points

Discussing infertility with your spouse is not just an obsession, it's a necessity. As we have seen in previous chapters, many medical decisions must be made which, ideally, should involve the consent and agreement of both spouses. These include

Watch Out!
If either you or your spouse feel at this point that you don't really want to have children after all, and that you're just going along with infertility treatments to please your partner, see a family or individual therapist right away.

Bright Idea
Ask your partner to watch TV shows or movies with you that deal with infertility or adoption. They can be just the ice breaker you need to get a discussion going on these topics. But, don't push it.

everything from which doctor to see, to when to change doctors, to trying IVF, to stopping treatment and pursuing adoption.

Infertility forces couples to confront issues and make decisions they never thought they'd have to make. They must talk to each other about these issues to avoid making decisions based on false assumptions.

These might include the meaning of family, the significance of children to a family, and the importance or irrelevance of having a biological connection to a child. All these areas are issues that can either bond a couple or cause conflict, depending on how much they agree or disagree with each other.

Here are some questions you should ask yourselves and each other:

- What is more important to us, becoming pregnant or becoming parents?

- Are we giving in to pressure from our parents or in-laws to produce grandchildren?

- Are we willing to sacrifice anything—money, the marriage, and so on—in order to achieve a pregnancy?

- Can we love a child who is not biologically ours?

Infertility requires constant evaluation and reevaluation of the situation to determine how much you can take medically, emotionally, and financially. Be sure also to ask each other—and ideally your doctor—the following questions every few months:

- Should we change doctors?

- Should we consider third-party reproduction?

- Can we afford this?

- Should we stop reproduction?

- Should we consider adoption or child-free living?

While these questions can lead to arguments, they can also lead to a better understanding of your own and your spouse's feelings and beliefs about these very important issues. Remember, it's not so much the answers to these questions that are important; over time, you and your spouse are likely to change your minds on some of these issues. The main thing is to talk to each other and keep the lines of communication open. When each partner is open to discussing infertility and his or her feelings, it tends to bring the relationships closer together.

In the next few chapters, we'll go into more depth about each of these important issues.

Fertility rights

We saw what can go wrong in a relationship as a result of fertility problems. Now let's see what can be done to set things right.

Not having children allows you to do things together you probably won't be able to do very often if you have children. Doing special things can also help keep your marriage happy, exciting, and alive. And you won't have to worry about child care or paying a baby-sitter.

- Take a vacation from infertility treatment and scheduled sex.

- Take a *real* vacation: Go somewhere that doesn't allow children, such as a honeymoon-type resort or health spa. This will help you realize there is more to life than children.

- Go to a romantic city, such as Paris, Venice, or the place you went to on your honeymoon or first date.

- Go to an exotic spot, such as Bali or Tahiti.

- Go on an adventure vacation where children are unlikely to be, such as a hiking, biking, or rafting trip.

- Go to the movies. Not those cutesy G or even PG movies, but romantic, sexy, R- or even X-rated movies. Not only will you be less likely to see children, the movies will most likely be about adult topics.

- Eat out in romantic, child-unfriendly restaurants.

- Eat in: have an adults-only dinner party at your home. Choose the couples carefully so discussions won't revolve around children or infertility. One way to do this is to have a gourmet pot-luck and wine-tasting dinner party.

- Plan a romantic evening alone with your spouse at home or in a hotel. Have a delicious dinner with wine and then watch a romantic or X-rated video.

Long-term effects

Infertility is likely to have some lasting effects on your marriage, both good and bad. Some couples do, in fact, split up as a result of infertility. Said one woman whose marriage was breaking up, "After five-and-a-half years of temperature charts and trying and anticipation, infertility really caused stress in the marriage and we're breaking up. Not just because of infertility, but it definitely contributed."

How you resolve your fertility problem, the options you ultimately choose—or don't choose— will certainly have an impact on your relationship. The good news is that infertility can bring you closer

> ❝
> The only thing worse than infertility for your sex life is having children!
> —David, a fifty-year-old editor and father of twins.
> ❞

together rather than pull you apart, especially if you follow the advice in this chapter and seek help when you need it.

Infertility can help couples gain a deeper understanding of and new respect for their partners:

> I think our relationship is stronger, our mutual respect for one another is greater, our love is certainly deeper, and it's a whole different relationship than when we started. And probably a much better one. Going through this process put a real strain on the marriage. But I can't imagine another thing happening in our marriage that we wouldn't be able to deal with, having survived and experienced this together.
>
> —Gail, a thirty-four year old speech teacher

Many couples feel that by confronting their fertility problems together and finding mutually satisfying solutions, marriages can be strengthened, and the effects can last for years. Ten years after her infertility experiences the following woman, who adopted two children, said: "We feel like we came through a storm and we're closer for it. We've gone through things that other couples never have and survived. That brought us closer together. We no longer take anything for granted with ourselves or our kids."

Just the facts

- Your sex life will change, but not forever.
- Women obsess about infertility more than men, but it doesn't mean men don't care.
- Involving your spouse in your infertility treatment can actually help strengthen your marriage.

GET THE SCOOP ON...
Deciding who to tell ▪ Handling insensitive
comments ▪ Dealing with pregnant friends ▪
Coping with infertility at work

Chapter 13

Living and Working in the Fertile World

I t's not only your marriage that's likely to be affected by infertility. Your relationships with friends, relatives, and co-workers can also be affected. Even the decision of when and how to tell others about a fertility problem is a very personal and sometimes difficult one. Many couples, understandably, are hesitant to tell friends and relatives. Some only tell others when they have to, such as when they are hospitalized after a miscarriage or for a surgical procedure.

Coming out

Deciding to tell others about your infertility is not always easy. Many people feel infertility is stigmatizing, embarrassing, and too personal to discuss with others. Some may want to discuss it with others, but their partners object. Most often, it's the male partner who finds it uncomfortable if the infertility problem is made public—many men feel threatened by infertility because they associate it with impotency. For them, talking to others about infertility is tantamount to admitting having sexual problems, even if this is not the case.

Disclosing your infertility, therefore, is a very personal decision that each couple, and each partner, has to make individually. It may help to ask yourself the following questions:

- What can I gain by telling that person?
- What are some of the possible negative ramifications?
- How would my partner feel if I told that person?
- Is that person likely to hear about our problem from someone else?
- Can I trust that person to keep our fertility problem confidential?
- Is that person sensitive and likely not to make upsetting remarks?

If you do come out and tell people about your fertility problem, it's hard to anticipate their reactions. Everyone has his or her own personal baggage about reproductive issues. Some will respond with sympathy, some with indifference, and some with embarrassment. Said one woman, a psychiatric social worker, "I went slowly telling people. I did total psychosocials on everyone before I told them, and I only told people who I knew would give a very supportive response. But it didn't always happen." Some are pleasantly surprised by how supportive their friends and relatives are when they mention about their fertility problems. Said one man, "I had been afraid to tell them partly because they have never been supportive of anything that I have ever done in the past. I was afraid they'd blame me for it that I would be seen as defective." It turns out that his mother had assumed they didn't want children. So when he told her they were having fertility problems, it was a big relief, and she was very supportive.

Strained relations

While many infertile couples find their friends and relatives very sympathetic and supportive, others complain about insensitive and unsupportive responses. One man describes what happened when he told an old friend: "I told him we were having fertility problems and he said that when he wanted to get his wife pregnant, he'd knock her up right away! I was really pissed off. When they did finally try, he turned out to have a major fertility problem. What poetic justice!"

But even comments that may be well-intended can hurt. In fact, you may find that there is very little anyone could say that you would find comforting. If the listener is too sympathetic, you may feel patronized. If, on the other hand, the listener makes light of your problem, and says, "You'll see, it'll all work out" you may see that person as unsupportive and insensitive.

Unsolicited advice

You may find that one of the most irritating things is when you receive unsolicited advice from friends and relatives, or even strangers. They might give you advice on everything from what doctor to see, to what fertility drug to take, to what sexual position is best. How do you handle this? It's probably best to thank them for their interest and say that you've already researched the subject and have carefully chosen a doctor whom you trust, and that you're taking your doctor's input about fertility drugs (and

Watch Out!
If you let others know about your infertility, you open yourself up to unsolicited advice, unwanted pity or even insulting remarks. On the other hand, if you don't tell someone, you open yourself up to being questioned over and over about when you're going to have children.

sexual positions). That if you need their advice later on, you'll be sure to call them.

Insensitive comments

You might find it even more annoying when the advice and remarks imply that the infertility is somehow your own fault. These comments might include: "Just relax and you'll get pregnant," "Take a vacation and you'll get pregnant," or "Adopt and you'll get pregnant." Although there is no scientific evidence for supporting the notion that stress is a major cause of infertility—and that a vacation or adoption will cure it—this is one of the most persistent myths about infertility.

Another thing that might drive you up a wall is when people make negative comments about having children, such as, "You're crazy to want kids; kids are a pain." Remember that your friends and relatives mean no harm by these comments, which are intended to comfort you. But remarks like these can really hurt.

Family gatherings can present a real challenge. There are always nosy relatives asking you questions. But insensitive questions and comments are not limited to relatives. Friends, as we have seen, can be incredibly insensitive and annoying as well.

Some people feel it's best to ignore these comments. Others find that the best way to handle these comments is by anticipating them and preparing retorts ahead of time. You can pretty much anticipate that your prying Aunt Sadie will say something like, "When are you going to stop being selfish and make your mother a grandmother?" and your Cousin Charlie will say something obnoxious such as, "Obviously, you guys don't know how to do it right. Want me to give you a lesson?" You might, for

Bright Idea
Try role playing with your partner and take turns being the one who makes the insensitive or obnoxious remark. The other has to come up with a good retort. This can be an extremely useful, not to mention enjoyable exercise.

example, say to Aunt Sadie: "We very much want a family but we're having fertility problems, and it pains me to talk about it." As for Cousin Charlie, you can laugh it off, walk away or say, "From what I hear, you wouldn't know where to begin."

Depending on how you feel about such people, and your future relationship with them, your retort can be polite, humorous, sarcastic or blunt. Many people prefer the blunt approach because it acts almost like shock therapy, and tends to stun and silence the person. One woman tried several approaches until she found one that worked for her:

> At first when people asked me if I was going to have children, I used to say, "We're trying." Later I just said, "We're infertile." And then I got to the point where I would say, "I'm barren." I did it on purpose, because when you say that you're trying, they ask you four thousand questions, but when you come out and say, "I'm sterile" or "I'm barren," they just shut up!

No news is good news

Most women with fertility problems are hypersensitive when it comes to anything to do with pregnancy, especially the pregnancy of others. Finding out about the pregnancy of a friend or relative can be especially disturbing. How the news is conveyed can make a difference. The following woman described what happened when she was awakened at night by a phone call from an older cousin who already had two children:

> My cousin said, "I just wanted to let you know before you heard from your mom, I'm pregnant." And I said, "Oh, congratulations. You must be really excited." I was totally

appropriate, but it was really hard for me. When I got off the phone there was sweat dripping down my arms. Later I realized how angry I was at her. She didn't have to phone me up at night. She could have written me a letter three days before she told the family…it would have been much better for me to read it so I didn't have to react. Because what am I going to say to her? "You b****! Don't you have enough already?"

While the pregnancy of a friend or relative may be the last straw, not being told about a friend's or relative's pregnancy can also be devastating. It may make you feel patronized and even more inadequate and vulnerable than you already felt. The thought that your friends find it necessary to protect you from the truth implies you're incapable of handling it, and can make you understandably furious. Said one woman: "There were people in the family who became pregnant and I wouldn't be told about it, and that really started driving me crazy. I felt that people shouldn't make the decision for me."

The fertile earth

Seeing mothers with their small children—whether you know them or not—can be an upsetting experience for infertile women, especially women who have had miscarriages. You may, therefore, want to avoid gatherings and places where pregnant women, babies, and toddlers may be present. It's not just their presence that can cause problems; these mothers and about-to-be mothers may not understand your lack of enthusiasm about their condition or children.

While being around babies and small children is hard for many, you will probably find that the hardest situation to bear is being around pregnant

> **"**
> Infertile couples should avoid events that they can foresee are tailor made to devastate them.
> —Barbara Eck Menning, Founder of RESOLVE
> **"**

women. Infertile women seem to have, as one woman put it, tunnel vision for pregnant women. Because of this, they tend to feel that the whole world's pregnant but them. Being among pregnant women often makes infertile women feel like failures. You may ask yourself why you can't succeed at something these other women seem to do with ease.

Someone else's pregnancy can cause feelings of jealousy, rage, inadequacy, guilt, and even hatred in infertile women. As a result, many infertile women have violent fantasies toward pregnant women, such as stabbing them in their bellies. Said the following woman, "A pregnancy was devastating to me—it destroyed me. I didn't want anything to do with pregnant women. I had fantasies of them having miscarriages, or stillborn or deformed babies. I wanted their pregnancies to fail so that they would be failures like I was." After a while, her husband also started having the same feelings, with some exceptions: "I wanted to punch pregnant women right in their big fat bellies. But I also felt happy when someone who had really struggled with infertility became pregnant. They were more deserving."

Some women are confused or embarrassed by these feelings. Said one woman, "I feel that I have a personality flaw, that my misfortune shouldn't color the way I relate to other people. But it does. I can't stand being near pregnant women. It does me in."

If you have these negative feelings and violent fantasies about pregnant women, remember that you're not alone. And fantasies can't cause harm. Even some men harbor these hostile feelings. Seeing a friend's pregnant wife can make an infertile man feel inadequate and pose a challenge to his masculinity.

To go or not to go

One sure-fire way to avoid these negative, hostile feelings is to avoid being around pregnant women if at all possible. If this sounds anti-social or weird to you, ask yourself, "Why should I put myself in a painful situation in which I have nothing to gain?" Protecting yourself from pain is not selfish, it's sensible.

Holidays such as Christmas, Hanukkah, Thanksgiving, Easter and Passover can be especially painful times for infertile couples. These are holidays that families celebrate together and are often very child-centered. It's virtually impossible to avoid the topic of having children at such occasions. They're also difficult to avoid, unless you have a really good excuse. So if a holiday or other occasion is coming up that you'd love to avoid, plan to take a vacation at that time. Being away is one excuse most people understand.

Probably the worst social situations for most women with fertility problems are baby showers, christenings, and other celebrations revolving around babies. Having to observe, and, even worse, participate, in the celebration of a pregnancy or new baby can be emotionally traumatic.

When you get an invitation to such an event, it may seem like a no-win situation—if you don't go, you may feel guilty. If you do go, you'll probably regret it because of the emotional pain it causes you.

Realistically, if you don't go to your friend's shower, it won't be the end of the world. After all, the party is about her and her baby, not you. She'll be so distracted by the party, the gifts, and everybody else, she probably will hardly notice your absence. Ask yourself, is it worth several hours of

Bright Idea
Because of strained relationships with the fertile world, you may find it easier to pursue friendships with other infertile couples. If you don't know other couples in your situation, you'll meet them by joining RESOLVE or other infertility support groups.

your emotional pain just to spare a friend a brief moment of disappointment?

If you're having trouble deciding whether or not to go to a baby shower, child's birthday party or other potentially painful event, ask yourself these questions:

- Is my presence essential?

- Will my absence really make a difference and ruin the event?

- Will the guest-of-honor suffer more by my absence than I will by my presence?

If you decide not to go, don't feel guilty about it. Going through infertility, perhaps more than most other diseases, requires that you protect yourself emotionally. The following woman described what happened when she went to her niece's first birthday party right after her second miscarriage:

I felt like, well, it's my sister. But when I stepped in the house I knew I had made the wrong decision. I was crying inside and just holding myself together. That's all I could do. It was dumb of my sister not to think it through; I think I would have. She had lots of mothers there with their babies. I decided I would never go through that again. It's my life, and it's too painful. I feel right now that I come first. I will not subject myself to people who are pregnant or have small children. If they don't understand, it's their problem, because I don't care right now. But that will pass. And if those friendships don't last, I don't care.

If possible, you should take care not to hurt the other person's feelings. As we said earlier, being out of town is probably the best excuse. If you can't get away, it may be best to be honest with your friend.

Moneysaver
Get a few friends to chip in to buy a baby gift. The gift will be nicer, you can save money, and you can get someone else to do the shopping for you.

Watch Out!
If you don't go to a baby shower or some other event, be sure to send a lovely gift and thoughtful note. Not to do so would probably add insult to injury in your friend's mind.

You can simply explain that you're in the midst of infertility treatment, and that while you're thrilled for her, you're unhappy with your situation. That being at a baby shower with a lot of people would make you extremely uncomfortable, and you're sure that she would understand. If she doesn't understand, she's not a good friend.

The good news is that you won't feel this way forever. Once you resolve your infertility—through a pregnancy, adoption, or decision to remain child-free, you most likely won't continue to be plagued by these hostile feelings toward pregnant women. Said one woman who adopted a baby, "Adoption brought an immediate and instantaneous relief to all these feelings of wanting to kill, take out a knife and stab every pregnant woman." And another woman described how she and her husband were flying home with their newly adopted baby, when a pregnant woman got on the plane: "I turned to my husband and said, 'She's pregnant and we've got ours!' It was really a nice feeling."

Also, if you do choose to continue your quest for a child—through a pregnancy or adoption—you and your long-awaited child will likely be the guest of honor at least one of these celebrations. And if an infertile friend doesn't want to go, you'll know just how she feels and let her off the hook.

Pregnant co-workers

As we have seen, you might become upset by being around pregnant friends, relatives, and even strangers. But these are situations you can potentially avoid. The problem becomes even more complicated when you have no choice, such as at work, and the pregnant woman is your co-worker, or worse still, your boss. You have to act professionally regardless of whatever feelings you may have of jealousy or hostility. And you certainly cannot avoid going to work.

Having to work with pregnant women can put a tremendous strain on your relationships with them—relationships that normally require objective professionalism.

At work—as in social situations—some people think it is best not to tell infertile women about co-workers who are pregnant. But this usually backfires since a pregnancy cannot be hidden for long. One woman, an assistant manager of a boutique, was extremely upset because her boss did not tell her that she was pregnant. What made it worse for her was that all the other employees were told, even the part-time ones. "I was the last person at work she told, so I was very angry with her. I said, 'I really think you should have told me—even if knowing would upset me—if for no other reason than because I am your assistant manager.'"

Job Interference

Women undergoing infertility treatment have many other work-related issues to deal with besides pregnant co-workers. Infertility can mentally and physically interfere with your work. There are times, for example, when you'll have to call the doctor from your job for test results or for specific instructions about medications. It may be difficult to find a private phone so that you won't be overheard.

It's especially difficult to concentrate on your work and carry on as usual when you get distressing news. Hiding your reactions and emotions is also not easy, as this graduate student discovered:

My doctor said to call him for the results of my second pregnancy test at three o'clock. I was in

Work can be an oasis from infertility.
—Beth, a social worker

Unofficially...
In the 1950s, doctors attributed infertility to women's pursuit of higher education. In the 1990s, they claim that much of infertility is the result of women pursuing careers rather than motherhood when they're in their twenties and early thirties.

the middle of interviewing a woman for a research paper and couldn't find a private phone, so I used one in the room. The nurse told me my hormone levels weren't rising as they should be, indicating a possible miscarriage. I started to shake and cry. I was really embarrassed and couldn't complete the interview.

Regardless of whether or not you have a private office, there are times when you may not be able to hide your emotions. The following teacher wound up having to tell her co-workers about her fertility problem: "There are times when I'm in my office and I'm crying or I have my head down and I'm hysterical. One time, however, I fell apart during a meeting and began to cry, so I had to tell them why."

Telling women you trust at work about your fertility problem can be helpful for some. But it's not always an option. Many women feel strongly about keeping their infertility a secret on the job.

Risky business

Many career-minded people find that infertility has a dampening effect on their enthusiasm for their jobs. Job performance can be adversely affected and careers put on hold, making career advancement—and satisfaction—extremely difficult. Said the following woman, an editor: "I've done very bad work in the last six months. I've barely been functioning. I'm no longer committed to my job. My work has gotten sloppy. The kind of work I do is creative, but when I'm depressed nothing is generated."

Diagnosis and treatment often require that a woman take time off from work for doctors' appointments. Many women complain that juggling work schedules and doctors' appointments is very disruptive and stressful, as this urban planner discovered:

> I haven't been able to work fulltime ever since the beginning of this. How can you, when you're taking off for this and that and the other thing, and going three times a month for artificial inseminations, and then this time for blood tests and that time for postcoital tests? I don't know how anyone can work full time and actually do all these tests, and then take off for a laparoscopy here and surgery there.

Because most people do not want employers and co-workers to know about their fertility problems, getting away from work—especially when it involves leaving early or missing important meetings—can be very difficult. "I had to lie all the time," said an executive. "It was tremendous pressure.... And I always felt guilty about it."

Taking time off for many doctors' appointments doesn't usually sit well with bosses, and raises the issue of whether or not you should tell them about your fertility problem. Admitting to being infertile is also an admission of planning a pregnancy. You may be legitimately concerned that the knowledge of your planned pregnancy could jeopardize your job. Many employers are upset when employees become pregnant because pregnancies cost companies time lost to maternity leave and money spent on insurance benefits. As a result, it can cost you your job. Although this constitutes discrimination and is illegal, unfortunately it does happen.

However, if you don't tell your boss or supervisor, he or she may wonder why you're leaving work and going to the doctors so often, possibly even worrying that you have a life-threatening disease that

Bright Idea
Check to make certain that if you try to get insurance coverage for your infertility treatment through your company insurance that they won't disclose your condition to your employers.

Unofficially...
If you lose your job because of infertility treatments or think you're being discriminated against for this reason, contact your State Attorney General's Office.

you are trying to conceal. You have to weigh all the pros and cons very carefully about disclosing your infertility status at work.

If your job involves travel, you have the added difficulty of not only fitting in doctors' appointments, but scheduled sex as well. One woman, a publisher, turned down one job in favor of a less desirable one because the first job would have required travel during ovulation. But another woman, a public relations executive, was lucky enough to work for a company that would fly spouses in for "conjugal relations," which she carefully planned to coincide with her ovulation.

You can work it out

Every job situation is different, as is every boss. When making work and career-related decisions, you have to weigh many factors and decide what's realistic, appropriate, feasible, and ultimately best for you and your career. Here are a few ideas that may work for you:

- Ask for a flexible work schedule that would allow you to periodically come in early and work late, or vice versa.

- Ask if you can work part-time for a limited period of time.

- Ask about working at home. With home computers and the Internet, more and more people are able to work at home successfully.

- Try to schedule your appointments during lunch hour or on weekends whenever possible.

The waiting game

As we have seen in earlier chapters, infertility involves a lot of waiting...waiting for doctors' appointments, test results, ovulation, an open slot at an IVF program, an adoption to come through, and on and on. As a result of all this waiting, many people have to, or at least believe they have to, put their lives on hold.

For many women, it's very often their careers that they put on hold while they wait for a pregnancy or baby that may or may not appear. They may not look for new opportunities or new jobs because any month now they may conceive. They may postpone major career moves or turn down great jobs just to stay in a job they may hate but find convenient, as did the following woman, a lawyer:

I kept expecting to get pregnant, and that's why I've kept this job. I don't like what I do, and I need to go job hunting and get a new job. On the other hand, if I get pregnant, I'm in a wonderful position because I can take time off. I can walk to work and would be four blocks away from my baby. If I'm going to have children, I'm working at the perfect place. So I keep delaying doing anything about it

By postponing positive career moves, you can wind up without either the job or the child of your dreams. The following physician took a non-prestigious job at a city hospital because, as she explained, "I thought that if I had a child it would be a really good job for me, but the job sucks, and I don't have a family. So now I'm angry at myself because I never should have made a decision based on something I had no control over."

Working through your problems
While infertility often has a negative effect on work and careers, many women find their jobs and careers help them deal with their infertility

Moneysaver
When considering changing jobs or staying where you are, it may pay to choose the job with the best infertility insurance coverage.

Timesaver
If your doctor doesn't have early morning or evening hours, you might want to ask the doctor to make an exception and see you once in awhile before or after work. If he or she refuses, you may want to switch to a more accommodating doctor.

problems. They find that their work helps keep them sane while going through the process of infertility treatment—that being able to throw themselves into their work and careers helps them forget about infertility, at least during working hours. Said one woman, a teacher, "One of the things that really has surprised me when going through infertility treatment was how much my work meant—how much a support and a lifeline it became."

Work is also a place where your worth is determined by hard work and achievement, not by whether or not you pass a pregnancy test. For some, work also helps to compensate for not having a baby, as this fund raiser discovered:

> The result of all my frustration and disappointment was that I got more involved in my job. It was a way to try to forget. I worked longer hours. I wanted to be productive. I wanted to produce a baby but I couldn't so I decided to produce a body of work. I just worked harder and harder, and was very successful. So it was nice. It paid off.

The type of work you do may also have some impact on both the way you cope with infertility and the way you cope with your job. While some people with fertility problems may find working with small children difficult, most seem to derive pleasure from it. Said one woman who worked with young children:

> I think I have an advantage working with children—it does take a certain amount of maternal feelings, even though it's on a professional level. It's enjoyable and I'm in an enviable position. I think it's more enjoyable for me than it would be to be an aunt or visit a friend's child. When I have these kids, they are *my* kids.

Keep in mind that you have a lot to gain by getting involved in your job. It can be a positive distraction, give you a sense of accomplishment, and help you feel in control over your life. Make the most of it and it will probably pay off professionally and financially.

Infertility can also have a positive effect on your career in unexpected ways. For example, some people, especially those in the helping professions who come in contact with people with fertility problems, find that their experiences with infertility help them deal more empathetically and effectively with their clients. "I've been able to help a lot of people pursue adoption or pursue infertility treatment," said an internist who ultimately adopted two children. "Not that I would wish an illness upon a doctor or other medical professional, but I think illnesses or physical problems help people be better doctors, nurses, or whatever."

Infertility can also affect someone's career choice. Some put so much time and energy into infertility that they decide to make a career out of it. For example, one woman, a career counselor who adopted a child, started a successful side business in counseling women on adoption. Another woman, a social worker who was president of a local chapter of RESOLVE, broadened her practice to include infertility and adoption counseling after she adopted a child. And many of the books about infertility and adoption, including this book, are written by people who have had personal experience of infertility.

Just the facts

- You can't anticipate anyone's reaction when you tell him or her about your infertility.

Watch Out!
Even though part-time jobs make it easier to fit in doctors' appointments, they may not be great for your career. Not only do they pay less, they tend to be less secure, less prestigious, and less likely to carry medical insurance than full-time jobs.

- It's normal to dislike being around pregnant women.

- Infertility can interfere with your job and career.

- By getting more involved in your work you will probably fare much better emotionally and financially than if you allow infertility to interfere with your career.

GET THE SCOOP ON...
Common emotional reactions to infertility ▪
Stress and infertility ▪ How support groups can
help ▪ Finding an infertility counselor ▪
Childfree living

Chapter 14

Surviving and Resolving Infertility

Infertility is considered a major life crisis for good reason. As we have seen in the past two chapters, infertility can negatively affect marriages, sexuality, interpersonal relationships, and careers. And, like all major life crises, infertility has serious emotional consequences for the individuals involved. Most couples feel they're on an emotional roller coaster, with ups and downs that seem to follow those of their temperature charts. If you ask couples with fertility problems what's the worst part of their ordeal, most will say without hesitation it's the emotional toll it takes on their lives. As one women put it, "The physical pain of surgery is over in a few days, but the emotional pain lingers on and on."

A multitude of losses

Barbara Eck Menning—founder of RESOLVE, the national organization for people with fertility problems—described the predictable emotional responses most people have to infertility: surprise, denial, isolation, anger, guilt, a sense of unworthiness, depression, and grief. These feelings are mainly due to the myriad losses a person with fertility problems suffers—the loss of control over one's life, the loss of a normal sexual relationship with one's spouse, and perhaps most importantly, the loss of the dream of having a child of one's own.

Loss of control

Loss of control is especially hard to accept for those who are used to being in control over their lives. Many talk about how, until they experienced infertility, they always felt in control. As a result, they're not used to failure, like the following woman, a teacher:

> I always accomplished what I wanted. I wanted my own apartment, I had it. I wanted my own life, I got it. I wanted to support myself in a style to which I had become accustomed, I had it. I wanted boyfriends, I had them. I wanted to get married, I got married. All of a sudden, a major thing, and I'm not getting it. I cannot believe it. It never occurred to me that I wouldn't get what I wanted.

Infertile men and, probably more so, women, also tend to experience a loss of control physically as well as emotionally. It can be a general feeling of their lives being out of control, or a more specific feeling of the physical loss of control over their reproductive lives, or both.

The physical loss of control can be especially difficult for those who are used to being in control of their bodies. They may, for example, have spent years controlling their fertility by carefully choosing and using contraception in an effort *not* to get pregnant. Now they find that control of their fertility is out of their hands.

When they feel that their bodies are betraying them, some people may try to compensate by taking control in other ways. Men may try to make their bodies appear more masculine and take up sports or bodybuilding with a vengeance in an effort to regain control. Women, too, may focus excessively on their bodies. As one woman put it, "I felt very unhealthy; my body wasn't doing what it was supposed to do. So I joined exercise programs and I joined weight-reducing program. This was all because I wanted to control my body, which was out of control."

Loss of self-esteem

Feeling out of control of your life can profoundly affect your self-esteem. Whether infertility primarily involves failure to impregnate your partner, failure to conceive, or failure to carry a pregnancy to term, infertility ultimately is the failure to become a mother or father, at least biologically. As a result, your self-image and self-esteem may suffer. "It's an ego-battering experience. I don't feel as pretty, and I certainly don't feel as fertile or as feminine," said one woman. People with fertility problems use words like inadequate, incomplete, flawed, defective, and damaged goods to describe themselves.

Loss of positive sexual identity

Many men see infertility as a negative reflection on their masculinity. For them infertility spells impotence. They equate fertility with virility. Women, too, often have a similar reaction and equate fertility with femininity. As one woman explained about her self-identity:

It's a reflection on my womanhood. I don't feel very womanly because my image of being a woman is to be a parent, a mother. I measure

Unofficially...
RESOLVE was founded in 1974 by Barbara Eck Menning in her home in Belmont, Massachusetts. She and five other women with fertility problems sat around her kitchen table and decided to start the organization to help themselves and others cope with infertility. The membership now exceeds 12,000.

myself a lot against other women whom I see with children and with careers, and with family life. And somehow I don't feel as good as they are.

Men do not carry any outward signs of their fertility or infertility, but women do—the pregnant belly is proof positive of being fertile. While not being pregnant doesn't necessarily tell the outside world you're infertile, many women do associate being a complete woman with pregnancy and biological motherhood.

Not being able to do what most other women can do—become pregnant and give birth—can distort a woman's sexual identity. Said one woman, "Sometimes I feel like I have a caricature of a woman's body. That it's sort of too feminine on the outside and it's no good on the inside."

When they don't conceive and, therefore, don't feel feminine, some women try to compensate by changing their external appearances. Some attempt to regain control over their bodies by losing a lot of weight. But, as we mentioned earlier, being excessively thin can interfere with conception. Others change the way they dress. "For a long time I really did feel less of a woman," one woman admitted. "I went through a period of wanting to look very, *very*, feminine. I stopped wearing pants. I let my hair grow long." But her behavior didn't last very long. She resolved her feelings of inadequacy and came to the following realization: "Not being able to have a baby doesn't make you any less womanly than having a baby makes you more womanly. What it is to be a woman is really socially, not biologically, defined."

To help you separate the ability to reproduce from masculinity and femininity, keep in mind that hundreds of thousands of men and women are voluntarily sterile. They choose to have vasectomies and tubal ligations—whether or not they've ever had children. In fact, men who have vasectomies tend to be considered quite "macho." And women who've had their tubes tied are certainly not considered unwomanly. Nonetheless, these men and women are totally sterile.

Some people are able to use their experiences with infertility to gain more insight and a deeper understanding of what it really means to be a man or woman, and a mother or father. They realize, like the woman above, that neither the ability to reproduce nor a biological connection to a child is necessary to adequately fulfill those roles. In fact, one woman said she felt that infertility actually made her feel *more* like a woman. "I really have had to come to grips with what it means to be a woman," she explained. She was able to come to the realization that the physical processes of pregnancy and childbirth were not what defined womanhood or motherhood.

Mourning your losses

Resolving the emotional issues surrounding infertility and coming to a realistic understanding of motherhood, fatherhood, and parenthood doesn't come easily. First, you need to accept that you're infertile. That involves going through a period of grieving for the many losses you suffer because of infertility. This doesn't mean that you'll never conceive or that you're at the end of the road and giving up. It just means that you acknowledge your condition.

Grief and mourning—and the tears that often follow—can be cleansing and healing. Grieving can help you come to terms with your infertility. Once you grieve about your losses, you can better make rational decisions not only about what to do next, but how and even if you're going to build a family.

Because of the losses it involves, many experience infertility as a death—the death of the dream of possibly having their own children and the death of children who might never be. The fertile world doesn't always understand this type of death and the need to mourn. As one woman poignantly explained, "It's not as if an actual person has died. So you can't get the kind of support you'd like, as you would if someone died. I don't know how to explain to people that this child in me, who never existed, died."

For those who have had miscarriages, the equation of infertility and death is even more real. But even though miscarriage is actually the death of a fetus, some people, including doctors, don't see it as such. They don't understand the depth of the couple's despair. Couples who have miscarriages are often told that miscarriage is nature's way of getting rid of a mistake, and they could always get pregnant again. Telling a couple who just experienced a miscarriage that the child they conceived was nature's mistake can add insult to injury. To them miscarriage is the actual death of their child, and treating it like a death, not a mistake, helps them cope and carry on. In fact, many couples have private services to help them mourn their lost child. Some find that burying items such as baby booties or performing other rituals can be especially helpful in recovering emotionally from this trauma.

Survival strategies

As you can see, people react to infertility in many different ways. There are also many different coping mechanisms available to help people deal with the

Unofficially... Some therapists call themselves infertility counselors because they see infertility patients as an educated, affluent, and untapped market. As with all health professionals, you should check their credentials and their experience.

various emotional crises of infertility. Some of the most common ones are religion, therapy, and support groups.

Religion

Some men and women with fertility problems find religion a major source of support and consolation. They may find the spiritual meaning of religion or the familiar rituals comforting and helpful. While some may turn to organized religion and prefer to worship as part of a group at a church, synagogue, temple, or mosque, others seek solace in a more personal, inward religion and prefer to be pray alone silently. Some may pray for a pregnancy and child, and some use prayer to help them resolve infertility in other ways as this woman did:

> I felt that I should try to be more religious, more accepting. I pray a little more, a little harder and more sincerely to try to be more accepting of what will be—just accept what God has destined for me. I've never prayed for a baby. To this day, I've never prayed, or lit a candle, or done a novena for a baby. I have prayed for strength. God knows we need a lot of that going through this process. I've prayed for insight to make good decisions for us.

Turning to religion for support, strength, and guidance may be a new experience for some. They might be quite surprised to find themselves being religious for the first time, as did the following woman, who had always regarded herself as an agnostic and viewed religion as a crutch:

> I became more Jewish about this for a while. I thought that would help. I was wearing a chai around my neck for a year because that was a symbol for life, and I thought if you wore a chai

Unofficially...
Recently, researchers at a leading metropolitan medical center reported several cases of post-traumatic stress disorder (PTSD), which is commonly seen in people who survive wars or natural disasters—in women experiencing infertility. They advised doctors to be on the look out for PTSD in infertile women and to be vigilant in monitoring them.

you'd get pregnant. Going to Israel was another part of the Jewish year.

And some may develop a religion of their own design to suit their own spiritual needs. For example, one woman who was born Jewish and became an atheist said that when things got really bad, she went to a church, lit candles and spoke to Jesus. "It helped because I just felt like I was trying basically to get a feeling that there was something outside myself helping me to cope with this," she explained.

Finding support from others

Many infertile people turn to their spouses, friends, and family for support and comfort. It's not unusual for them to reach out to different people at different times, as this woman described:

> There were times when my husband was an anchor for me, and at other times my mother has been very good. At other times it's been my nephews—just seeing two normal children playing and having a marvelous time is a reaffirmation of what you want to do when you get discouraged. At other times it's been work. Being able to say I have other things that make me important. Other times it's been me. And permeating this whole experience has been a religious orientation.

Self-help organizations and support groups

Virtually everyone with a fertility problem needs others to talk to who can relate to their situation. But it's not always easy to find people who can really understand what you're going through, much less talk about infertility. As we saw in previous chapters, spouses aren't always available, able, or approachable to discuss infertility issues. And, unfortunately, those in the "fertile world" often lack empathy and

Bright Idea
If possible, interview a few infertility counselors before settling on one. Choose carefully since he or she can have a profound effect on both your emotional life and the decisions you make around the issue of infertility.

understanding about the subject. However, self-help organizations, such as RESOLVE, and the support groups are often run by these organizations and by fertility clinics.

RESOLVE and similar organizations can be extremely useful for anyone with a fertility problem, whether the person just beginning treatment, is in the midst, or is thinking of stopping. Becoming a member of RESOLVE, and/or joining an infertility support group, is probably the single best thing you can do for yourself to help you deal with the social, emotional, and medical issues related to infertility.

RESOLVE—the largest self-help organization for people with fertility problems in the United States—is a national, non-profit, volunteer association that has over fifty chapters across the country. It offers referrals to fertility specialists and therapists and has a telephone hotline, information brochures, reading lists and other relevant resources. Most local RESOLVE chapters offer monthly meetings where doctors or therapists who specialize in infertility speak. They also typically offer support groups for men, women, and couples that meet on a regular basis and are typically led by a mental health professional.

People join RESOLVE and other infertility self-help or support groups for a variety of reasons. Some want to get information about infertility treatment or fertility specialists. But most do so for emotional support. They may not know anyone else with a fertility problem and want to meet people going through the same difficulties. One woman said she joined a support group at the fertility clinic she attended because her husband had forbidden her to discuss their problem with anyone else and she found it intolerable to be so isolated. Some

Moneysaver
RESOLVE members can use both their local and national hotline and support lines, and get valuable help and information over the phone. It only costs $45 to join, considerably less than it would cost to go to a private therapist.

people join because they're curious to see what other infertile couples look like and act like. They're usually amazed that everyone looks normal and healthy—just like they do.

Overcoming barriers to joining

Some people are reluctant, however, to attend a RESOLVE meeting or join a support group. If you're one, it may help to think about what you're afraid of. In Chapter 13, we discussed a similar situation—being hesitant to disclose your infertility to friends and relatives because you fear what they might think about you and say to you.

In both situations, you're not only labeling yourself infertile, you're admitting to others that you have a fertility problem. But there's one big difference: Everyone in the support group is in the same boat! They, too, suffer emotionally and physically, have been the victims of insensitive remarks, and have had to live in the sometimes cruel fertile world. It's very unlikely that they'll be judgmental. On the contrary, they can empathize with you. A bonus of being in a support group is that members often share doctors' names, good and bad experiences, and valuable information about treatments and adoption. You can feel free to laugh and cry together. So you have a lot to gain from being with others with similar problems, and nothing to lose.

By now, you may be eager to join RESOLVE but find that your partner isn't. Women in general tend to be more receptive to joining support groups and self-help organizations than men. So many women take the first step and join a group, and sometimes their spouses follow. But sometimes they don't. RESOLVE is still primarily run and attended by

Bright Idea
If your partner is resistant to going to a RESOLVE meeting, try to get together with some other RESOLVE couples for drinks or dinner before a meeting. It might be just the ice-breaker you need to get a reluctant person involved.

women, although more and more men attend meetings and support groups each year.

For those who do attend meetings or support groups, most find it comforting, reassuring, educational, or helpful in some way. Even spouses who are dragged there tend to "come around"—literally and figuratively—after they get over their initial anger or embarrassment.

Support groups fulfill needs that spouses, friends, relatives, therapists, and doctors often cannot. Many say that a major benefit of support groups is finding others like themselves. It's not just an issue of "misery loves company." It's finding people who are nonjudgmental and with whom you can share your problems. Said the following woman:

> I was astonished to find there were a lot of others like me. I had never discussed this with anyone for a lot of reasons. It was all inside me. The only one I spoke with or cried about this with was my husband. I guess it became too overwhelming and I felt we couldn't help each other anymore. So, I started going to meetings.

As we said earlier, a major benefit of being in a support group and/or self-help organization is that you become extremely knowledgeable about many of the medical aspects of infertility. You get the chance to listen to and have your questions answered by guest speakers who are often top fertility specialists in your area. You can also hear first-person accounts by their fellow patients.

Support groups are especially helpful when you're faced with resolving infertility through egg or sperm donation, surrogacy, adoption, or childfree living. And just being with others struggling with the same issues can be helpful.

> **"**
> It was a relief to meet other people and also to find out that my reactions to the whole thing were not as bizarre as I was being told they were by my husband.
> —Elaine, a psychiatrist married to a psychologist
> **"**

Seeking professional help

As good as support groups are, they aren't for every-body. Also, there may not be one in your area. So if you feel you can benefit from emotional or psychological help, and support groups are not the answer, you may want to consider seeing a therapist. Seeing a therapist does not mean you need to be in long-term therapy or analysis.

Individual psychotherapy and psychological counseling are common ways people get help dealing with short-term crises, as well as long-term problems. You might just need help in getting over the emotional crisis of infertility, and help in sorting through the pros and cons of the various options available to you.

And, as we discussed in Chapter 12, you may decide that seeing a marriage counselor or family therapist can be helpful in resolving the infertility-related issues—and other pertinent issues—in your marriage.

If you're not sure whether or not you should see someone, the Mental Health Professional Group of the American Society of Reproductive Medicine (ASRM) provides the following list of symptoms or situations that *might* indicate that you should see a therapist.

- Persistent feelings of sadness, guilt, or worthlessness
- Social isolation
- Loss of interest in usual activities and relationships
- Depression
- Agitation and anxiety
- Increased mood swings

- Constant preoccupation with infertility
- Marital discord
- Difficulty concentrating and remembering
- Confusion about treatment options
- Change in appetite, weight, sleep patterns
- Considering third-party reproduction (donor egg, donor sperm, donor embryos, surrogacy)
- Increased alcohol or drug use
- Thoughts about suicide or death

Keep in mind that you're likely to have experienced many, if not all, of these symptoms at some point in the course of your infertility diagnosis and treatment. But you may need the help of a therapist if these symptoms persist over an extended period or if any of them are extreme or interfere with your life and daily functioning.

Finding an infertility counselor

If you've decided you should seek professional help for infertility, you now have to find the best person for you and your situation. There are many different types of mental health professionals who might consider themselves infertility counselors. They can be psychologists, psychiatrists, psychiatric social workers, family therapists, marriage counselors, nurses, and pastoral counselors. The main thing to remember is that they should be professionally trained and have credentials in their field of mental health. In addition, it is very important that they have specialized training and knowledge in the field of infertility.

Infertility counselors should be specifically trained to deal with the emotional—and even some physical—aspects of infertility. Infertility counseling, however, is a relatively new profession, with no uniform training, so it's often up to the individual therapist to seek out adequate training.

Many infertility counselors are mental health professionals who have experienced infertility themselves. Ideally, an infertility counselor has undergone some training in reproductive medicine by working closely with fertility specialists, in a fertility clinic, or by attending postgraduate medical as well as psychological courses. It's up to you to find out.

One good way to find an infertility counselor is through your local chapter of RESOLVE. You can ask your doctor or fertility clinic if they work with an infertility counselor or if they can recommend one in your area. You can also contact the ASRM's Mental Health Professional Group mentioned above, and ask for their membership list. The membership list will not, however, give you information on a member's qualifications—you'll have to check that out for yourself. But ASRM membership at least shows that infertility is a field of special interest to.

Here are some questions you should ask about the infertility counselors you're considering:

- What degree do they have and where did they get their training in therapy? Your therapist should have a minimum of a master's degree, usually in psychology, social work, or counseling, from a reputable graduate school.

- Are they licensed to practice therapy? Being licensed as a mental health professional guarantees that a therapist has had postgraduate training.

- What infertility experience have they had? Have they worked closely with a fertility specialist or in an ART program? If so, for how long? Make

Watch Out!
If you're seeing a therapist who objects to or does not support your joining RESOLVE or another support group, find a new therapist.

sure the therapist has worked with a reputable doctor or program, or has had some training in infertility.

■ What percentage of their practice is infertility? It's probably better to see an infertility counselor who devotes at least half-time to treating people with fertility problems.

■ What professional organizations do they belong to? Besides being a member of ASRM's Mental Health Professional Group, the therapist should be a professional member of RESOLVE. Membership in these organizations is an important indication of the therapists interest and dedication to the field of infertility. Belonging to other mental health organizations is also important.

■ Have they personally experienced infertility? This question is tricky. In general, therapists don't divulge information about their personal histories. But many make an exception in the case of infertility counseling. While it's not necessary that a therapist has had a fertility problem to help couples cope with the emotional aspects of infertility, it can be helpful. Adequate training, experience, and sensitivity are probably more important. But a personal history of infertility can also be useful in helping clients. *As long as therapists are able to remain objective,* they may be able to draw on their own experiences to help you make decisions about various treatment options, adoption, and even childfree living.

As you can see, it may not be easy to find a therapist who's trained in the physical and emotional

Moneysaver
Make certain the therapist you're seeing is fully licensed in your state. Your insurance company may not reimburse you for sessions unless he or she is.

Watch Out!
Be aware that some counselors who've had infertility problems themselves might be living out unresolved issues through you. Rather than being objective, they may give you advice based on their own bad experiences.

aspects of infertility and can truly understand infertility in a nonjudgmental way.

Traditionally trained therapists

Traditionally trained therapists can be very helpful for many emotional problems, including some of those related to infertility. However, most therapists are not trained to deal with the unique issues infertile individuals or couples face. Therefore, they may not adequately understand the emotional and medical aspects of infertility that people with fertility problems face.

In fact, one of the most frequent complaints people with fertility problems have about traditional therapists is that they, like many uninformed people in the fertile world, tend to believe that stress, ambivalence, and other psychological factors are major causes of infertility. By emphasizing stress, these therapists are, in effect, blaming the victim. This can be not only painful and counterproductive, but confusing—especially if you're being treated for a specific, diagnosed physical problem.

Stress and infertility: cause or result?

Being told that you're infertile because of unconscious factors or stress can make you feel guilty and more depressed—not to mention more stressed—than you already are. One therapist told a woman who had a diagnosed ovulatory problem, "Your mind is very powerful. It could be that this is a case in which the harder you try the more difficult conception becomes." Her therapist had, like many who do not understand infertility, jumped to the conclusion that ovulatory problems were the result of psychological problems.

As we mentioned in Chapter 2, even if you have unexplained infertility, there is little evidence that stress is a significant cause. Some evidence does exist that stress can interfere with ovulation in certain cases. But it's virtually impossible to determine if, and when, ovulation problems may be the result of stress. In addition, the woman above, like most women being treated for ovulatory problems, was taking fertility drugs. So even if her therapist was correct and stress was a causative factor, it wouldn't matter since fertility drugs more than compensate for the possibility of emotionally induced anovulation.

And, remember, millions of women living under extreme emotional, physical, and financial stress manage to conceive with ease. In fact, in some of the poorest countries with the worst living conditions, such as India, China, and parts of Africa, overpopulation—not underpopulation—is a major problem.

That's not to say you shouldn't try to relieve stress. Stress is probably the most common emotional side effect of infertility. Relieving stress in any way possible is a good idea. In fact, although it might seem contradictory to what we said above, relieving stress might help you conceive, at least indirectly. The less stressed you are, for example, the more likely you'll want and have sex. Depending on the cause of your fertility problem, the more frequently you have sex, the better your chances to conceive. And the less stressed you are, the more likely you'll be to make positive decisions about your infertility treatment and other options.

Deciding enough is enough

At some point, the emotional, physical, and financial stresses of infertility may get to be so

Moneysaver
Massages are one of the best stress busters you can find, but they can be expensive. Rather than pay for one, you and your partner can give each other massages. It's also a nice way to be physically close without the pressure to conceive.

Unofficially...
According to Childless By Choice, a national organization for childless couples, an estimated 10 percent of couples in the U.S. today are childless, and many of them are childless by choice.

overwhelming that you say, "Enough is enough!" Or you may have pursued all the options medically and socially acceptable to you and your partner. If you're at this point, you have three choices:

Take a break. You may want to take time off from treatment, and, at least temporarily, get on with your life. Taking time off from treatment gives you time to reflect on your situation and review your options more objectively. It also can be physically helpful, since taking fertility drugs and/or undergoing invasive treatments can take their physical, as well as emotional and financial toll. Many doctors insist their patients stop taking fertility drugs for several months to give their bodies a chance to get back to normal. In fact, it's not unusual for patients to conceive during a break from fertility drugs. Again, this is not because they're under less psychological stress (although that may be a positive side effect), but because their bodies are under less physiological stress from treatment.

Revisit your other options. You may decide to reconsider one of the donor or surrogacy options, or adoption. What seemed out of the question to you or your partner a year or even a few months ago may now not seem like such a bad idea. This is when being in a support group can be extremely helpful. Being able to talk to others who are now struggling with these issues, or have done so in the past, can give you invaluable insights as well as information.

Start doing more research on the options that seem most appropriate and appealing. It might help to first reread Chapters 9 and 10 in this book about third-party solutions, including adoption. Then turn to the Appendix of this book to find Internet sites, books, and organizations that can provide you with more information about these options.

Consider childfree living. You may decide that you want to put infertility totally behind you and get on with your life. This, for most couples, means choosing to be childfree. Unless, of course, you already have children living with you. In that case, you may choose accept your family as it is and stop trying to have or adopt another child.

Childless by chance...or choice

Many infertile couples who previously considered themselves involuntarily childless make a decision to be childfree. Choosing to be childfree should and can be a positive decision. In fact, that's why we prefer the term *childfree*, an active term with positive connotations to *childless*, a passive term with negative implications.

Choosing to be childfree, like choosing to adopt, is a positive decision that means you are taking control over your life and moving on. While you didn't have control over your previous state of childlessness, you can now take control.

And choosing to be childfree doesn't mean giving up. After all, living a childfree life is what you've probably been doing for quite a long time. Before this whole infertility mess happened, you and your partner were probably very happy together without children. You can continue to be happy together... just the two of you. Michael Carter—who co-authored *Sweet Grapes: How to Stop Being Infertile and Start Living Again*, with his wife, Jean Carter—wrote the following about their decision to remain childfree:

> Childfree means that we have taken the strength we found in our struggle with infertility and turned that strength toward making our lives good again. It means taking advantage of

> 66
> Contraception was our declaration of independence from the cycle of hope and despair and for us the final step in being childfree.
> — Jean and Michael Carter in *Sweet Grapes: How to Stop Being Infertile and Start Living Again* (p.27)
> 99

the benefits that can come from not having children.... To me...the most important part about the childfree option is that it offers a message of hope to all of us who are infertile: even if you don't end up with a child, you and your spouse still have the potential for a happy, productive life together. It says that two can also be a good size for a family.

—quoted in RESOLVE Fact Sheet, "Childfree Decision-Making," by Merle Bombardieri.

Talking points

Couples want children for many reasons, some reasonable, and some not so reasonable. In trying to decide if you should continue to pursue pregnancy, seriously look into adoption, or remain childfree, you might want to go back to basics and ask yourself why you want to have children. Understanding your motives—both the rational and irrational ones—can help you make the right decision for yourself and your spouse. Ask yourself, and your partner, the following questions about why you want to become pregnant and/or have children.

- Are you pursuing this to please your spouse? Your parents? Your in-laws? While your spouse's wishes are key, the wishes of your parents or in-laws should not influence your decision. If your spouse, however, wants children and you don't (or vice versa), you have a serious problem and may be helped by seeing a family therapist or marriage counselor.

- Do you want a child in part because you want to relive your happy childhood? Or conversely, are you trying to rewrite your unhappy childhood and right what your parents did wrong? Whether your childhood was happy or sad, remember, no two children or childhood experiences are ever alike. Your child will be a totally different person and will grow up in a totally different family environment. Probably your parents, like most, decided to raise you differently from the way their parents raised them! And, as much as we'd like to, we can't guarantee our children will have a happy childhood.

▪ When you picture your child, do you picture a sleeping infant, cuddly baby, or a chubby-cheeked toddler? If so, remember, the early years go by very quickly and parenthood goes way beyond babyhood. Can you picture yourself parenting a precocious pre-adolescent or a temperamental teenager? Or what about a handicapped child? There is no guarantee that your child will look like one of the babies in the Gap commercials.

▪ Are you trying to fill a void? Do you want a child because you're bored with your life or job? Raising a child will certainly keep you busy—it's time-consuming and can be all-engrossing. But, as any parent will tell you, much of parenting is boring and tedious. And there's no paycheck at the end of the week. Remember, while you can quit a job you don't like, you're a parent for life. Also, it's unfair and unrealistic to expect a child to fill a void in your life.

▪ Do you want children so you won't be alone when you're old? By now, you should be well aware of the fact that things don't always go as planned. Having children certainly is no guarantee that you will live to a ripe old age. And even if you do, you're children may have other plans.

There are no right answers to the questions above. They may all apply to you to some extent. However, if any one of them is your *primary* motive, perhaps it should give you pause.

The need to nurture

You probably wanted children in the first place because you liked being around them and/or felt a maternal or paternal need to nurture. Childfree couples can certainly have children in their lives, be they nieces and nephews, children of friends, or children in their community. In fact, volunteering to work with children, especially underprivileged children, is a wonderful way to help both them and yourself.

You can volunteer to:

- Be a reading (or math) tutor at your local school.
- Be a Big Brother or Big Sister.
- Be a mentor in an after-school program.
- Be a scout leader.
- Be a little league coach.
- Be a Sunday school teacher.
- Work with homeless children.
- Work with children with AIDS.
- Work with handicapped children.
- Be a foster parent.

Another way to fulfill your need for nurturing is by bringing pets into your life. They require care, nurturing, and affection. And you get plenty of affection in return.

Bright Idea
Try to spend some afternoons, evenings, or weekends, if possible, alone with friends' or relatives' children of various ages. It will give you a more realistic sense of what it's like to have children.

Ambivalence

It's normal to feel ambivalent about any major decision. In fact, you or your partner might have been
ambivalent about having children in the first place.
But once you got caught up in pursuing pregnancy,
you might have lost sight of that original ambivalence, and the reasons for it. If you or your partner
were initially ambivalent, it may help to recall some
of the reasons for that initial ambivalence.

Childfree living is obviously not for everybody. If
you're uncertain—and you probably are since
you've devoted so much time, energy and money
into trying to have children—you should read as
much about the subject as you can. Try to find a
support group for childfree couples or couples seriously considering this option. Join chat rooms on
the Internet. Try to observe and talk to as many
childfree couples as you can. Ask them about the
issues that concern you. Said the following woman
about her recently widowed aunt and uncle:

> My aunt and uncle were one of the happiest
> couples I've ever known. Because an ectopic
> pregnancy ruined her tubes, my aunt could not
> have children. However, they loved surround-
> ing themselves with their nieces, nephews, and
> friends' children. But more than that, they
> loved being together and were totally devoted
> to each other. Up until the day my uncle died,
> at the age of eighty-two, they acted like newly-
> weds. Does my aunt have any regrets? Only one.
> That she outlived her beloved husband.

Remember, if you have a child, there's no turning back, but if you do make a decision to remain
childfree, it's not written in stone. You can change
your mind down the road and look into other

Unofficially...
Research studies
have shown that
childfree couples
are just as happy
as couples who
have children.

Bright Idea
Make a list of the pros and cons of having children and the pros and cons of being childfree. Although many items will be the same, you may uncover some interesting pros and/or cons by looking at the issue from both points of view.

options, especially adoption and even foster parenthood. Most couples, however, who do make the decision to remain childfree are happy with that decision and stick with it. While they may have moments of regret, we all have those moments about every decision we make, including the decision to have—or not to have—children.

Just the facts

- Mourning your infertility-related losses can help you resolve your infertility and get on with your life.

- Most psychotherapists are not trained to deal with the emotional aspects of infertility.

- Joining RESOLVE or some other support group is one of the best ways to help you survive and resolve your infertility.

- Childfree living is an option you may seriously want to consider.

GET THE SCOOP ON...
Treatment costs ▪ Insurance legislation ▪
Understanding your policy ▪ Reimbursement
strategies

The Financial Side of Infertility

Chapter 15

The diagnosis and treatment of infertility has made major strides over the past 20 years, so that couples need not simply resign themselves to childlessness. But getting the necessary treatment paid for is still extraordinarily difficult. According to RESOLVE, two-thirds of America's childless couples need not stay that way, but for the costs of treatments.

These costs can be high, depending upon the treatment required. The actual charges for treatment of infertility varies from state to state, and from treatment to treatment, but by breaking the treatment programs down into component parts, it's possible to come up with an estimate of the kind of money you're looking at having to pay.

An infertility treatment cost breakdown

No matter what form of treatment you ultimately decide upon, you will have to undertake an initial consultation. This may cost anywhere from $150 to $400—where you live makes a big difference.

315

Timesaver
Gather all your insurance documentation before you go in for your first appointment, once you've settled on a doctor. The facility's office manager or billing supervisor will be better able to help you work out the best way to approach your insurer for total or partial reimbursement if you've got your policy information at your fingertips.

Medical care of all types tends to be far more expensive in major urban centers than elsewhere in the country. Chapter 3 provides you with several tips on how to keep your consultation costs down.

After your initial consultation with the doctor of your choice, you'll have to undergo a basic workup (see chapter 4 for details on the workup). The workup itself consists of a variety of tests, from screening for infectious disease to ultrasound and laparoscopy. Each test adds to your overall costs, as table 14.1 shows:

TABLE 15.1: AVERAGE COSTS ASSOCIATED WITH THE STANDARD INFERTILITY WORKUP

Test Type	Cost
Blood test	$200-$600
Hormone testing	$180-$1500
Semen analysis	$45-$120
Ovulation test	$0 if done by basal body temperature charting; $40-$90 if done with an ovulation induction kit.
Ultrasound	$75-$200
Ultrasound (pregnancy)	$175-$375
Endometrial biopsy	$75-$375 for the biopsy; $50-$150 for lab analysis
Post-coital test	$45-$190
Hysterosalpingogram	$200-$400
Cannulization of fallopian tubes	$500-$800
Laparoscopy	$450-$600 for anesthesia; $1,400-$3,500 for hospital stay; $1,000-$4,000 for surgeon's fees
Hysteroscopy	$1,000-$2,500

Sometimes additional blood tests may be required—to measure hormone levels during ovulation or during the luteal phase—and these will add from $45 to $100 to your bill, per test. And do keep in mind that your particular case may not require every one of the tests included in the basic workup. It's best to go into the process knowing what the possible costs are, however. As table 14.1 shows, the total can range from $2,850 to $8,100, or more.

If the basic workup fails to disclose any abnormalities in your reproductive functions or those of your partner, further testing is indicated. These advanced tests (discussed in detail in Chapter 4) can run from $200 to $400 for a hemizona assay or a sperm penetration assay. Antibody testing can cost from $75 to $100 per test, and an immune series may be run, which can costs from $1,000 to $1,800. Obviously, in both the basic workup and in the advanced testing phase of your infertility treatment, it may be necessary that some tests be run more than once, further increasing treatment costs.

Medication costs

In addition to the cost of the tests themselves, medications may be required. For ovulation induction— the most commonly recommended treatment for infertility—the drug clomiphene citrate (CLOMID or SEROPHENE) is prescribed, at an average cost of $20 to $55 per ovulatory cycle. In some cases, clomiphene citrate is replaced by, or prescribed in conjunction with, human menopausal gonadotropin (PERGONAL, HOMEGON), or other medications. These can be very expensive, especially if purchased in the U.S. PERGONAL and METRODIN (a urinary follicle stimulating hormone frequently used with clomiphene) can cost as much as $75 per dose in the U.S., whereas in Mexico the cost per dose can be as low as $17.

The difference in drug prices can have a major impact on your total cost of treatment. Since you will need to take anywhere from 15 to 40 doses during a single ovulatory cycle, the U.S. cost of the medication can range from $788 to $2,120, whereas the same drugs purchased in Mexico would cost from $255 to $680.

Intrauterine insemination (IUI)

Should your doctor recommend that IUI be performed during the ovulation induction cycle, you'll be looking at a further series of charges. These are broken down in Table 15.2:

Unofficially...
The basic elements of the IUI procedure will run somewhere between $180–$510 per cycle, but this total does not take into account any additional booster shots of hCG, which will add about $40 per shot.

TABLE 15.2: IUI COSTS PER OVULATORY CYCLE

Procedure	Purpose	Average Price Range
hCG injection	triggers ovulation	$20-$40
Laboratory preparation of sperm	prepares sperm for insemination	$75-$250
IUI procedure	insemination of sperm into the uterus	$45-$200
Progesterone suppositories or daily progesterone injections	luteal phase support	$40-$120

Monitoring costs

In addition to medication, infertility treatments require that your physician monitor you through the ovulatory cycle. The costs that you might incur at this point are highly variable. It depends on how many ultrasound scans (at $75-$200 per scan) or blood tests (at $45-$100 per test) one would need.

When surgery is required

If you and your doctor have determined that you will need surgical intervention, the costs of infertility treatment rise dramatically. Depending on the condition requiring treatment, total fees for surgical intervention can range from $3,100 to $18,000. Table 15.3 gives a breakdown of these costs for common surgical procedures used to correct infertility:

TABLE 15.3: COSTS OF SURGICAL TREATMENT FOR INFERTILITY

Type of Surgery	Hospital Fees	Anesthesia	Surgeon's Fees
Hysteroscopy, myomectomy	$1,200-$3,500	$400-$600	$1,500-$4,000
Laparoscopy	$1,800-$5,000 (with laser, $2,300-$6,500)	$400-$1,000	$1,200-$4,000
Exploratory laparotomy	$4,500-$13,000 (includes OR and recovery)	$800-$1,000	$1,800-$4,000

Unofficially... Your doctor cannot legally suggest that you purchase your medications outside of the U.S. He or she is required to prescribe only drugs that have received FDA approval and are purchased within U.S. borders.

Surgical intervention is obviously more costly than outpatient procedures for a number of reasons. The most significant cost factors are surgeon's fees and the cost of the hospital stay itself, and the latter costs can really mount up if there are any complications that extend your stay. Unaccounted for in the cost breakdown is a further cost: the recovery time at home that may last as long as 6 weeks. If you're employer will not provide paid sick leave for an extended a period of absence, you must take into account the lost income you will incur as well.

Assisted reproductive technologies (ARTs)

The ARTs are the high-end infertility treatments. They are also, unfortunately, the least likely forms of infertility treatment to be covered by insurers. These technologies, discussed in detail in Chapters 8, range from in vitro fertilization (IVF) to gamete intrafallopian tranfer (GIFT) and zygote intrafallopian transfer (ZIFT). The cost is even further increased if your IVF treatment requires an egg donor or surrogate carrier.

GIFTs will cost as much as IVFs, and then some—they have the additional expense of egg

Unofficially...
Where you live makes a real difference in the costs of these procedures—a simple IVF can range from $3,500 to $11,000, and that's before you add in the costs of ovulation stimulating drugs.

recovery to consider as well. Table 15.4 provides a breakdown of the costs associated with ARTs.

TABLE 15.4: BREAKDOWN OF BASIC COSTS ASSOCIATED WITH ARTs, PER CYCLE

Procedure	Average Cost Range
IVF	$6,500-$6,800
Ovulation stimulating drugs	$2,000-$5,000
Embryo freezing	$100-$500
Embryo storage costs (often not charged for first year)	$10-$50/month
Frozen embryo transfer (with estrogen-progesterone preparation of the uterus)	$600-$2,000

When you add in the costs of involving a third party in your infertility treatment, the costs increase dramatically. At this point, legal fees are added to the medical costs, as are fees for medical and psychological screening of the surrogate. Finally, payments to the surrogate—insurance coverage, medical expenses, and delivery of the child—must be accounted for. The use of a surrogate gestational carrier can cost anywhere from $39,000 to more than $55,000. This is in addition to the costs of the IVF itself.

The great insurance debate

While it is relatively common for couples to need some form of help in overcoming problems of infertility (worldwide, one in every six couples of reproductive age experience fertility problems), it is decidedly *not* common for most of them to be able to afford treatment. Costs are high, and in these days of HMOs and coverage limitations, it can be extremely difficult to find ways to get the treatments you need without breaking the family bank. Some insurers refuse to cover any of the costs associated with infertility treatment. Others restrict their coverage to the basic workup, or cover only some of the available treatments. If your particular condition is not among those for which covered treatments are appropriate, your insurance is not going to be of much help to you.

When you combine the fact that different carriers offer different means of coverage with the difficulty most of us face when trying to understand the contract-legalese of most insurance policies, trying to figure out what you can count on for help in paying for treatment can be daunting. This is perhaps the biggest reason why an estimated 60 percent of all infertile couples never even explore treatment options.

Moneysaver
The cost breakdown for ARTs presupposes a single cycle—a circumstance that rarely applies to real-life treatments for infertility. A couple can typically expect to undergo ART therapy for at least two or three ovulatory cycles.

What's the problem?

The single biggest reason for the difficulty in finding appropriate insurance coverage for infertility treatment is that there are no real standards for it in the health insurance industry, and no state or federal agency standards for the regulation of coverage. Coverage disparities can be noted among insurers, as well as among states.

A few states mandate coverage for infertility treatment in one way or another. But "mandated coverage" means different things in different states. So-called soft mandates—the most common type—require only that insurance be available in theory—they do not require that it actually be provided. "Hard" mandates are a much rarer breed—they require that some form of insurance coverage be offered to the insurance consumer (that's you) as opposed to just the insurance buyer (your employer). But even where coverage is "hard" mandated, lack of enforcement has often meant that insurers feel free to delete it or deny payment. Only

Unofficially...
Only 19 states have any legislation that requires carriers to provide some form of infertility treatment coverage, and only 12 of these address coverage for ARTs.

two states, Massachusetts and Illinois, actually have put some teeth into their legislation.

A part of the problem is that, in the U.S., infertility is largely regarded as a non-necessity. The health insurance industry argues that the costs of covering procedures like IVF would price their overall coverage packages beyond the reach of most of the buyers of insurance—and the buyers are employers, not individual patients. In the insurers' view, infertility is not a disease—it doesn't threaten life or health—but rather a dysfunction. In addition, they tend to define the expensive, high-tech ARTs as "experimental" rather than as accepted medical practice.

Proponents of coverage for infertility treatment, on the other hand, strictly hold to a definition of infertility as an illness. The American Society of Reproductive Medicine takes issue with the definition of ARTs as experimental, citing a high live birth rate per IVF cycle (15 percent) that approximates the normal conception rate for healthy couples (20 to 25 percent).

The legal dimension

One route that has been taken to force coverage from employer-provided insurers has been to attempt to force federal legislation defining infertility as a disability. The Americans with Disabilities Act (ADA) of 1990 contains a provision that "requires reasonable modifications of policies and practices that may be discriminatory." This has been interpreted by some to mean that employers may be required to modify the insurance coverage they offer to include infertility treatments.

Breaking down the language of the ADA provision, the legal argument for coverage starts with the premise that health insurance is a significant "policy and practice" of employment: It is a standard benefit offered to workers, provided on a contractual basis. While there is no federal requirement that employers *offer* insurance to their workers, once insurance *is* provided, the employer is required to include coverage of disability conditions unless there is good cause for their exclusion. The limitation of coverage must be based on "sound actuarial data or other legitimate business or insurance justification," writes Gwen Thayer Handelman, associate professor of law at Washington and Lee University, School of Law. The denial of coverage, then, can be justified by demonstrating that providing it would be too costly fo the employer to bear.

This argument has implications for paying for infertility treatment on two counts, both of which lie at the heart of the debate between insurers and proponents of coverage. These are:

■ Is infertility a disability?

■ Is it too costly for employers to offer coverage for infertility treatment?

Both of these issues are currently being addressed in federal courts, and remain unresolved as yet.

Infertility as disability. The fundamental point of disagreement between insurers and proponents of infertility coverage is whether or not reproduction can be defined as a "major life activity." A disability, according to the ADA, must involve an impairment that impacts upon an individuals ability to engage in one or more major life activities. Unfortunately, the ADA never specifically defined what "major life activity" means. Walking, seeing, hearing, and learning are examples of such activities that have been accepted by consensus in the

Unofficially... Perhaps the hardest procedures to get insurance reimbursement for are the reversal of a voluntary vasectomy or tubal ligation. This is because the original cause of infertility is easily treated as the individual's prior choice—and thus in no way definable as a disease-based condition.

courts, but other activities, such as procreation, are still disputed. One side of the debate argues that major life activities are only those that have a "public, economic, or daily character" (*Bragdon* v. *Abbott*, a case challenging the right of an employer to deny dental coverage for a woman with asymptomatic HIV+ status). The other side argues that reproduction "falls well within the phrase" and is "central to the life process itself," (Supreme Court decision on *Bragdon* v. *Abbott*). The ultimate determination as to whether or not reproduction is a major life activity, and therefore that infertility qualifies as a disability, remains to be made.

Is infertility treatment too costly for employers to have to cover? Even if the determination is made that infertility is a disability and thus covered under the ADA, it is possible for employers to refuse to provide coverage for certain disabilities if providing it would be too costly. If the cost of providing coverage would constitute an "undue burden" on the employer, the ADA permits that it be excluded from benefits packages.

The insurance industry, and many employers, make the claim that it is indeed the case that infertility coverage would be too expensive. However, in 1993 a team of researchers provided a study for the Massachusetts Commission on Insurance. The study reviewed insurance data on infertility treatment collected by nine insurers, whose insureds, taken together, accounted for 65 percent of all privately insured people in the state. The researchers found that infertility treatment costs constituted 0.41 percent of the total medical expenses for the period under study (1986 to 1993). In dollars and cents terms, this works out to $1.71 per month per insured. The researchers concluded that there were no appreciable increased insurance costs to the consumer.

Until these two issues—infertility as disability, and the cost to consumers of providing coverage—are resolved, there is no likelihood of federally mandated coverage for infertility treatment. Proponents for coverage, most notably RESOLVE and ASRM, are actively involved in supporting cases that will provoke definitive court rulings supporting the right of individuals to secure infertility coverage.

The state-by-state breakdown

The twelve states with legislation that addresses the full range of infertility treatments vary widely to the degree in which they mandate coverage and enforce the laws that currently appear on their books. Perhaps the most favorable state for securing infertility coverage is Massachusetts; California, on the other hand, is far less helpful because enforcement of its mandates is lax. Here's a summary of the coverage mandated by legislation in the 12 states that address IVF procedures in their law.

- **Arkansas:** Health insurers providing maternity benefits are also required to cover IVF. HMOs, however, are exempt. The law stipulates that to qualify for coverage for IVF the insured couple must be able to show a 2-year history of unexplained fertility and the female's own eggs, and her spouse's own sperm, must be used in the procedure. The requirement of proof that unexplained infertility has lasted 2 years may be waived if the infertility is associated with endometriosis, fetal exposure to DES, blocked or surgically removed fallopian tubes (but not if

Watch Out!
Insurers and infertility treatment advocates profoundly disagree on the costs to insurers of offering coverage. You'll see studies cited by both sides, each offering a different perspective on the issue. Check the sources of the studies cited to see if they might to be biased by the opinions or objectives of the group that commissioned their research.

due to voluntary sterilization), or abnormal male factors. Insurers may impose a lifetime maximum payout of $15,000.

■ **California:** Insurers who cover hospital, medical, or surgical costs are required to *offer* coverage for infertility diagnosis and some infertility treatments, but they need not *provide* it, nor are employers required to include it in the package they offer to employees. Insurers are specifically exempted from having to provide IVF. If the employer is a religious organization, it is exempt from having to offer any coverage for treatments that are in conflict with the organization's ethical stance.

■ **Connecticut:** Coverage for infertility diagnosis and treatment, including IVF, must be *offered* but need not be *provided.* Employers are not required to include it in their coverage packages.

■ **Hawaii:** Individual and group health insurance plans, hospital contracts, and medical service plans that provide pregnancy-related benefits must provide a one-time benefit for outpatient costs related to in vitro fertilization, if and only if the patient meets certain conditions. The conditions include: only the eggs and sperm of the insured couple may be used; at least 5-years of unexplained infertility must be documented; other treatments covered by insurance have been tried and proven unsuccessful; the infertility is associated with endometriosis, exposure to DES, blocked or surgically removed fallopian tubes, abnormal male infertility factors are present. Treatment can only be performed at certain, specified medical facilities.

■ **Illinois:** Policies covering more than 25 people must include coverage for the diagnosis and treatment of infertility. Coverage is extensive, and includes four egg retrievals per lifetime. Coverage for ARTs (IVF, GIFT, ZIFT) has the following conditions attached: all reasonable, less expensive treatments have been tried and have been unsuccessful, and the facilities performing the procedure meet standards set by ASRM or the American Collete of Obstetricians and Gynecologists. Religious organizations whose teachings do not countenance infertility treatments are exempt from the requirement that they offer coverage.

■ **Maryland:** Health and hospital policies covering pregnancy are required to cover IVF, but HMOs and businesses with 50 or fewer employees are exempt from this requirement. The conditions for coverage include: only the insured couple's sperm and eggs may be used; less expensive treatments have been tried first and have been unsuccessful; the facilities meet ASRM standards; there is a 5-year history of unexplained infertility. If the insured also has endometriosis, exposure to DES, or blocked or surgically removed fallopian tubes, the other conditions need not apply.

■ **Massachusetts:** All HMOs and insuranc companies that cover pregnancy must also cover medically necessary expenses of infertility diagnosis and treatment. Mandated coverage is broad and includes IVF, GIFT, and ZIFT.

■ **Montana:** HMOs must include infertility services in their package of basic preventive health

Unofficially...
A legal mandate to *offer* insurance is not the same thing as a legal mandate to *provide* it.

care coverage. Non-HMOs are specifically excluded from this requirement.

- **New York:** Insurers are required to cover diagnosis and treatment of medically correctable conditions, including conditions that result in infertility. Specifically excluded from this requirement are reversals of voluntary sterilization, IVF, and other procedures solely intended to produce pregnancy.

- **Ohio:** HMOs are required to include infertility treatment in their package of basic preventive health service coverage. A $2,000 cap on the required coverage is imposed unless the infertility is associated with another condition, such as endometriosis.

- **Rhode Island:** Insurers covering pregnancy must also cover the diagnosis and treatment of infertility. Co-payments cannot exceed 20 percent of medical costs.

- **Texas:** Insurers must make it known to employers that coverage is available, but they need not provide it. For IVF coverage, the insured couple can only use their own eggs and sperm; other, less expensive treatments have been unsuccessful; the patient and her spouse can show a 5-year history of infertility. These requirements are waived if the infertility is associated with endometriosis, exposure to DES, blocked or surgical removal of fallopian tubes, or oligospermia. Religious groups whose beliefs are in conflict with the provisions of this law need not provide this coverage to their employees.

What's covered, what's not

In the absence of a coherent set of industry and federal standards requiring coverage for infertility therapy, couples seeking treatment are faced with a patchwork of policies, plans, and state laws. A 1996 study by Stacy Stove, reporting for Kiplinger Online (www.kiplinger.com/magazine/may96/inferti. html) provided the following data:

- 25 percent of traditional insurers offered some form of coverage for infertility treatment.

- 37 percent of HMOs offered at least partial infertility treatment coverage.

Some policies cover diagnostic procedures but won't pay for treatment. Some will cover low-tech treatments, and most refuse to cover such high-tech treatments as IVF. And even when treatments are covered, drugs are often excluded.

So, what to do if you're considering infertility treatment but can't handle the out-of-pocket expense? First, explore your insurance options. If your current plan provides little or no coverage, check to see if you can change carriers, and if there is one available to you that covers more of your costs. And by all means, take a long hard look at your treatment options. If you can't get coverage for the whole treatment regimen, break it down. Seek coverage for its component parts.

Type of carrier makes a difference

The amount of coverage available to you for your infertility treatment will depend upon the type of insurance plan you carry. There are four general types of insurance plans:

Bright Idea
Many states require that you document a long-standing (2 to 5 year) condition of unexplained infertility. Make sure you save all records of your treatment, from the very first consultation—the first time you receive a diagnosis—so you can address this question if your insurer raises it.

Unofficially...
Even if you live
in a state that
mandates infer-
tility coverage,
self-insurers are
normally exempt
from the terms of
the mandate.
Since large
companies are
generally self-
insurers, the
state mandates
do not apply
to them.

- Commercial companies: Aetna, Prudential: basic medical plan, major medical plan, or combo

- Non Profits: BlueCross/BlueShield: basic and major medical combo

- Self Insurers: employers who pay benefits directly: basic and major medical combo

- Provider Networks(PPOs)/HMOs: require primary care provider who'll authorize your use of a specialist. This type of insurer can be one of four types:

1. Staff Type HMO

2. Group Type HMO

3. IPA Type HMO

4. Network Type HMO

The first three types of plans generally have either a deductible (averaging about $250 to $500 per year) or co-payment (percentage of total) that you are liable to pay. The fourth usually imposes a co-payment obligation on its insureds in the form of a specific dollar amount that is payable by the insured at the time a service is performed.

Coverages offered will also vary by state, as well; and state laws often impose different requirements on the various types of insurers. Your first order of business in seeking help for covering the costs of infertility treatment is to determine whether or not your state has mandated infertility treatment coverage, the terms of any such mandate, the type of insurer that issued your policy, and the terms of your insurance coverage.

Decoding your policy

There has been a trend in recent years away from the legalese that once characterized all insurance policies, but the contracts are still difficult for most of us to understand. A common mistake made by employees is to confuse the "statement of benefits" they receive upon their initial employment with an actual copy of their policy. The Employee Retirement, Insurance, and Security Act (ERISA) requires your employer to provide you with a true copy on your request, but you'll probably have to go to your human resources department to pick one up.

Once you've secured a copy of your actual insurance contract, one that is dated for the current year and bears all necessary signatures, it's time to sit down and evaluate the language to determine precisely what kind of coverage you're entitled to. Here's a checklist of what to look out for:

☐ Exclusions. Check to see if infertility services in general, or specific treatments like IVF, are specified.

☐ Limits of Coverage. See if there are any specified limitations of coverage. Some policies have a total lifetime limit for all medical coverages, some may specifically place a cap on infertility treatments.

☐ Read through the specific terms of coverage. Some policies will cover "services to restore reproductive abilities" but exclude infertility treatments that seek to use artificial means to achieve pregnancy. This exclusion means that IVF and IUI won't be covered.

☐ Check the terms of coverage for diagnosis. Even if your coverage excludes infertility treatment but does not specify that diagnosis is excluded, you should be able to file claims for coverage of diagnostic testing and procedures—these can

Watch Out!
Don't assume that because coverage is issued in your name, you are the owner of the policy. Unless you are privately insured, the owner of the policy—the actual client of the insurer—is your employer.

make up one third of your total infertility therapy costs.

☐ Check your coverage for prescription drugs. If it specifies that all prescriptive drugs are covered, you may be able to get reimbursed even if your policy specifically excludes infertility *treatment.*

Once you've gotten a good sense of just what your insurance excludes, you're in a better position to start calculating how you're going to handle the costs of your infertility treatment. Keep in mind that while "infertility treatment" may be excluded, individual components of that treatment may not be. At this point you have to decide just how much to tell your employer and your insurance carrier.

What to tell your insurer

Because the actual owner of the policy that provides your coverage is your employer, you want to be careful about how much you disclose when you begin infertility treatments. This is especially true if your insurer places limits on your infertility coverage. Remember, your employer can generally change the terms of your coverage at any time simply by contacting the insurer and negotiating new terms or exclusions. If your policy currently provides favorable coverage terms for infertility, but your employer (or insurer) chooses not to accept the liability, tipping either one off on your plans to undergo fertility treatment might easily spur a quick change in coverages offered, and you might find yourself facing medical costs that you had blithely assumed were covered.

Mum's the word

There *are* benevolent employers who will willingly provide coverage, just as there are insurers who will pay for your infertility treatments, but unless you know for certain that this is true in your case, you need to take care to protect your financial interests. Until the legal climate has changed to more directly favor the patients over the interests of business, it is probably wise to be discrete about your treatment plans. This will require that you work with the financial advisor or office manager at your treatment center or clinic.

For example, your treatment can be billed as a single charge for the total services rendered—let's say, for an IVF. Your claim for coverage could quite easily be denied. However, claims for fees covering individual elements of the IVF procedure might easily be covered, if they are billed separately. Your clinic's office manager can prepare individual bills for your various blood tests and ultrasound tests, as they were broken out in the beginning of this chapter. Similarly, if your policy excludes IVF but covers treatment for the underlying causes of infertility, payment for much of the diagnostic treatment, and even the fertility drugs, might be offered without a protest.

Other creative cost-cutting options

If your current insurance carrier or HMO has very restrictive policies regarding the coverage of infertility treatment, and your employer provides a list of alternative insurance options, explore the terms of the other carriers on this list. It may be very much worth your while to switch plans to one more lenient in its coverage. Once again, however, make certain that you do this early on—preferably before you begin any infertility treatment and your employer learns that you're seeking such treatment.

Consider taking out a private health insurance policy. These are far more expensive than the insurance plan offered through your employer since you

Unofficially...
Religious groups are exempt from providing policies to their employees that cover treatments that conflict with the beliefs of the group. For many, infertility treatments fall in the "conflict" category.

foot the entire premium bill yourself, but if you know that you are likely to need one of the high-end ARTs, the greater coverage afforded by a privately negotiated insurance contract can easily offset the increase in premiums you'll have to pay.

As mentioned earlier in the chapter, you can achieve significant savings on some aspects of you infertility treatment simply by leaving the country. There is a marked difference in price for most infertility drugs, for example, once you leave the U.S. However, this is a cost-cutting option that you'll have to assume on your own—your physician is legally bound to prescribe only medications that the FDA has approved and that are purchased within the borders of the U.S.

Finally, if you have enough time to plan well in advance of seeking treatment, and you live in one of the states that provides no mandate for coverage (or fails to enforce mandates that have been passed by the legislature), you might consider relocating. Massachusetts has the most patient-friendly legislation mandating infertility treatment coverage, while California and Texas are extremely lax in enforcement of their laws, and 39 states have no protective legislation at all.

Just the facts

- The high cost of infertility treatment is the main reason that many couples don't seek help.
- Even if your insurance policy specifically denies coverage for infertility treatment, you may still be able to get many of the component tests and procedures covered if you file for them separately.

- Legal issues surrounding insurance coverage for infertility treatment are currently under hot debate in state and federal legislatures.

- Where you live and where you go for treatment can have a significant impact on both the cost of your care and the likelihood of your being reimbursed.

Glossary

acrosome reaction test test used to determine if sperm heads can actually undergo the chemical changes needed to dissolve an egg's tough outer shell and penetrate it.

adhesions scar tissue that attaches to the surface of organs.

AIDS (Acquired Immune Deficiency Syndrome) immune disease caused by the human immunodeficiency virus (HIV).

amenorrhea absence of menstruation.

aminocentesis procedure performed around the 16th week of pregnancy in which as small amount of amniotic fluid is removed and studied for chromosomal abnormalities.

ampulla trumpet-shaped area of the Fallopian tube near the ovary; also, a widening in the upper end of the vas deferens in which sperm are stored.

androgens male sex hormones.

andrologist medical doctor, board-certified in the diagnosis and treatment of male reproduction problems.

anovulation total absence of ovulation; menses may still occur.

anteflexed uterus a uterus that is tilted forward, and folds inward upon itself.

anteverted uterus a uterus that is tilted toward the front of the abdomen.

antisperm antibodies immunological reaction that causes a hostile environment in cervical mucus.

antisperm antibody measurement test performed to detect antisperm antibodies.

artificial insemination (therapeutic insemination) see therapeutic insemination.

aspermia absence of sperm and semen.

aspiration procedure in which follicles are retrieved from ovaries, and sperm are retrieved from the testes or epididymis by means of suction.

assisted hatching micromanipulation procedure using chemicals, mechanical techniques, or lasers, in which the outer surface of the embryo is thinned to help improve implantation.

assisted reproductive technology treatment methods related to in vitro fertilization and embryo transfer.

azoospermia absence of sperm in the seminal fluid; may be due to blockage or impaired sperm production.

basal body temperature body temperature which rises during the time of ovulation.

basal body temperature (BBT) chart record of basal body temperature over time to detect when ovulation has likely taken place. This is a crude test prone to error; its main advantages are its low cost and simplicity.

beta-hCG test blood test to determine pregnancy.

biochemical pregnancy (chemical pregnancy) a positive blood or urine hCG test, but one that does not continue to a clinical or on-going pregnancy.

biopsy surgical removal of a tissue sample for analysis.

biphasic pattern a distinct temperature elevation seen on basal body temperature chart.

blastocyst early stage of embryo development, usually occurring around day 7 after fertilization, at which time a fertilized egg loses its protective coating and is ready to attach in the uterine lining.

blastomere one cell of an early, multi-cell embryo.

bromocriptine (Parlodel) fertility drug taken orally; used to lower prolactin hormone levels and therefore allow ovulation.

capacitation change in a sperm cell that renders it capable of fertilizing an egg as it moves through the female reproductive tract.

CBC (complete blood count) routine blood test to determine the presence or absence of infection and/or anemia.

cervical canal an opening into the uterus which produces mucus that facilitates sperm movement.

cervical mucus secretions that are produced by the cervix; change consistency during the different phases of the menstrual cycle; during ovulation, cervical mucus becomes thin and watery to facilitate sperm movement into the uterus.

cervix the lower portion of the uterus projecting into the vagina; produces mucus that facilitates different steps during conception.

chemical pregnancy see biochemical pregnancy.

Chlamydia trachomatis organism responsible for chlamydial infection; considered a sexually transmitted disease, which may cause infertility and neonatal infections.

chromosomal aneuploidies   abnormal number of chromosomes.

chromosomes   rod-shaped bodies in a cell's nucleus which carry the genetic material (DNA).

cilia   hair-line projections found in the Fallopian tubes.

cleavage   early division of fertilized egg.

clinical pregnancy   pregnancy in which the fetus is shown to have a heart beat on ultrasound examination.

clomiphene citrate (Clomid, Serophene)   fertility drug, administered orally, used to stimulate FSH and LH production.

conception   fertilization of an egg by a sperm resulting in an embryo.

corpus luteum   special structure that forms on the ovary from an ovulated follicle and begins to produce progesterone to help the endometrium prepare for a fertilized egg.

cryopreservation   technique used to store cells, usually sperm, embryos, and eggs, in a frozen state for later use.

cryptorchidism (undescended testes)   condition in which the testicles do not descend properly into the scrotum during fetal development.

culdoscopy   a rarely used test in which a telescopic-like device is inserted through a small incision in the vagina to visualize the ovaries, the exterior of the Fallopian tubes, and the uterus.

danocrine (Danazol)   orally administered drug commonly used to treat endometriosis.

DES (diethylstilbestrol)   synthetic estrogen that had been thought to prevent miscarriage; responsible for some types of male and female infertility.

diagnostic hysteroscopy test in which a small telescopic-like device is inserted thorough the cervix into the uterus to examine the inside of the uterus.

diagnostic laparoscopy test in which a small telescopic-like device is inserted thorough a small incision in or near the naval to examine the abdominal and pelvic organs.

diethylstilbestrol see DES.

donor uteri see gestational carrier.

Down syndrome genetic disorder, caused by a chromosomal abnormality, which causes mental retardation, facial malformations, and other medical conditions.

dysmenorrhea painful menstruation.

dyspareunia painful intercourse.

ectopic pregnancy pregnancy in which the fertilized egg implants outside the uterine cavity (usually in the Fallopian tube, the ovary or the abdominal cavity).

egg donation third-party reproduction method in which eggs from a fertile woman are donated to an infertile woman for use in an assisted reproduction technology procedure.

egg retrieval procedure in which eggs are removed from an ovary for fertilization in the laboratory.

ejaculate seminal fluid expelled during orgasm.

electroejaculation process that can be used to stimulate the ejaculation in men who have been paralyzed below the waist.

embryo early stage of fetal growth.

embryo donation third-party reproduction method in which an infertile couple agrees to give extra or unneeded embryos to another infertile couple.

embryo transfer procedure in which an embryo produced through an assisted reproductive technology method is inserted into a woman's uterus.

endocrinologist medical doctor trained in the diagnosis and treatment of hormonal (endocrine) diseases.

endometrial biopsy procedure in which a sample of tissue is removed from the endometrium for analysis.

endometriosis condition in which normal uterine (endometrial) tissue is found outside the uterus; can cause painful menstruation and infertility.

endometrium uterine lining.

epididymis tightly coiled, tubular structure attached to the testicle, where sperm mature and are stored.

estradiol (E_2) hormone released by the ovary and produced by a growing follicle.

estrogen major female sex hormone produced mainly by the ovaries.

Fallopian tubes pair of narrow tubes that carry the egg from the ovary to the uterus.

female factor infertility used to describe infertility attributable to the female.

fertilization union of an egg and sperm.

Fertinex injectable fertility drug containing pure FSH used to stimulate the development and maturation of ovarian follicles.

fetal loss miscarriage and stillbirth.

fetal reduction medical procedure to decrease the number of fetuses within the uterus in a multiple pregnancy.

fetus developing human organism after the 9th week of pregnancy until birth.

fibroid noncancerous tumor found in the uterine wall.

fimbria fringed, finger-like outer ends of the Fallopian tubes.

FISH see fluorescence in situ hybridization.

fluorescence in situ hybridization (FISH) test that helps identify chromosomal abnormalities in fertilized eggs.

follicle tiny, fluid-filled structure on the ovary which contains and eventually releases an egg during ovulation.

follicle-stimulating hormone (FSH) hormone produced by the pituitary gland that stimulates the ovary to develop a follicle.

follicular phase first half of the menstrual cycle during which an egg-containing follicle develops.

FSH see follicle-stimulating hormone.

gamete male or female reproductive cell; sperm or egg, respectively.

gamete intrafallopian transfer assisted reproduction technology procedure in which eggs and sperm are placed in the Fallopian tubes.

gestation period of fetal development in the uterus until birth.

gestational carrier (donor uteri) a woman, not a genetic parent, who agrees to carry a pregnancy to term for an infertile couple.

GIFT see gamete intrafallopian transfer.

GnRH see gonadotropin-releasing hormone.

gonad male or female sex organs; testicles or testes in men, ovaries in women.

gonadotropin hormone that can stimulate the testicles to produce sperm or the ovaries to produce eggs.

gonadotropin-releasing hormone (GnRH) hormone released from the hypothalamus that controls the synthesis and release of FSH and LH from the pituitary gland.

Graves' disease see hyperthyroidism.

gynecologist medical doctor, board-certified in the diagnosis and treatment of diseases of the female reproductive tract.

hamster (sperm) penetration assay (SPA) test to determine whether sperm are capable of penetrating deep inside a hamster egg and fertilizing it.

HCG see human chorionic gonadotropin.

high-resolution scotal sonography or **venography** test to find varicoceles in the testicles too small to be felt during physical examination.

HIV human immunodeficiency virus, responsible for the development of AIDS.

HSG see hysterosalpingogram.

human chorionic gonadotropin (HCG)(Pregnyl/ Profasi) hormone, chemically related to FSH and LH, produced only when a fertilized egg reaches the implantation stage. Sometimes called the "pregnancy hormone." When given to a woman with a mature follicle, it induces ovulation.

human menopausal gonadotropin (hMG) (Pergonal/Humegon) an injectable hormone that contains both human FSH and LH and used to cause follicles to mature.

hydrocele fluid buildup in the scrotum.

hyperthyroidism (Graves' disease) excessive thyroid activity; increases the risk of miscarriage.

hypo-osmotic swelling test used to help predict whether sperm can fertilize an egg.

hypospadias deformity in which the urethra does not open at the tip of the penis.

hypothalamus a gland, located above the pituitary at the base of the brain, that sends hormonal signals to start the menstrual cycle.

hypothyroidism deficiency in thyroid function.

hysterectomy surgical removal of the uterus.

hysterosalpingogram (HSG) X-ray procedure using a contrast dye to evaluate the size and shape of the uterus and determine if the Fallopian tubes are open.

hysteroscopy telescopic instrument inserted through the cervix, to visualize the inside of the uterus and locate fibroids, polyps, scarring, and congenital deformities.

idiopathic infertility see unexplained infertility.

implantation embedding of the fertilized egg in the lining of the uterus.

infertility inability of a couple to achieve a successful pregnancy after one year of unprotected sexual intercourse.

intracytoplasmic sperm injection micromanipulation procedure in which an individual sperm is inserted into an egg.

intrauterine insemination (IUI) procedure in which washed sperm are inserted directly into the uterus.

in vitro fertilization (IVF) assisted reproductive technology in which eggs and sperm are collected (retrieved) and are placed in a dish in the laboratory for fertilization. Any resulting embryos are gently placed in the uterine cavity (embryo transfer).

IUI see intrauterine insemination.

IVF see in vitro fertilization.

Klinefelter's Syndrome congenital abnormality in males that causes sterility, secondary female characteristics, and possible mental retardation.

laparoscopy surgical procedure in which a telescopic-like device is inserted through a small incision in or near the navel to visualize the pelvic cavity, the ovaries, fallopian tubes and the exterior of the uterus.

laparotomy abdominal surgery.

leuprolide (Lupron)   fertility drug containing a GnRH analog which stimulates the female hormones initially, then suppresses FSH and LH secretion.

LH   see luteinizing hormone.

LH surge   dramatic rise in luteinizing hormone levels that culminates in ovulation.

luteal phase   second half of the menstrual cycle, ranging from ovulation to the end of menses or embryo implantation.

luteal phase defect   luteal phase with inadequate progesterone production in the second half of the menstrual cycle.

luteinizing hormone (LH)   hormone, secreted by the pituitary gland, that causes the ovary to release a mature egg.

male-factor infertility   term to describe infertility attributable to a condition in the male partner.

menopause   cessation of menstruation.

menstruation   cyclical, physiologic discharge through the vagina of blood and mucosal tissues from the nonpregnant uterus.

MESA   see microsurgical epididymal sperm aspiration.

Metrodin   injectible fertility drug containing FSH used to stimulate the development and maturation of ovarian follicles.

micromanipulation   procedures that allow working with a single sperm, egg, or embryo.

microsurgery   surgery in which microscopes, fine instruments, and microscopic sutures are used.

microsurgical epididymal sperm aspiration (MESA)   procedure in which sperm are removed from epididymis.

miscarriage   uninduced loss of a fetus.

Mittelschmerz sign mild pain in the abdomen on or about the time of ovulation.

monophasic pattern no distinct temperature elevation seen on basal body temperature chart.

morphology see sperm morphology.

motility see sperm motility.

myomectomy surgical removal of fibroid tumors from the uterus.

oligospermia low number of sperm in the semen.

oocyte egg, the female gamete or reproductive cell.

ovarian failure inability of the ovaries to respond to hormones and develop follicles.

ovarian hyperstimulation syndrome (OHSS) condition characterized by enlarged, painful ovaries and occasionally fluid accumulation; a possible side effect of ovulation induction.

ovary female sex glands in which eggs are formed.

ovulation release of mature egg from a follicle on the surface of an ovary.

ovulation induction use of fertility drugs to stimulation ovulation.

ovulatory phase time, usually around mid-cycle, when a mature egg is discharged from a follicle.

ovum egg released by the ovaries.

PCOS see polycystic ovarian syndrome.

PCT see postcoital test.

pelvic inflammatory disease (PID) pelvic disease usually caused by sexually transmitted or other infections and which often leads to infertility.

penis major male reproductive organ.

percutaneous epididymal sperm aspiration (PESA) procedure in which sperm are extracted from the epididymis.

percutaneous testicular sperm aspiration (TESA) procedure in which a needle is inserted through the scrotum, and sperm are aspirated from the testes.

Pergonal see human menopausal gonadotropin.

PESA   see   percutaneous   epididymal   sperm aspiration.

PID see pelvic inflammatory disease.

pituitary small gland beneath the hypothalamus that secretes many hormones, including follicle stimulating hormone (FSH) and luteinizing hormone (LH), which stimulate egg maturation and hormone production in the ovary.

polycystic ovarian syndrome (PCOS)   condition caused by an imbalance in follicle-stimulating hormones, in which the ovaries contain many cystic follicles; Stein-Leventhal Syndrome.

polymerase chain reaction (PCR)   technique that replicates specific DNA sequences many times for analysis.

polyspermia   fertilization of an egg by more than one sperm.

postcoital (Sims-Huhner) test (PCT)   microscopic evaluation of cervical mucus shortly after sexual intercourse to determine sperm quality.

preimplantation genetic diagnosis (PGD) technique that can be used during IVF procedures to test embryos for various genetic disorders prior to their transfer.

premature ejaculation   discharge of sperm from the penis prior to, or immediately after, entering the vagina.

primary infertility   infertility in someone who has never had children.

progesterone   hormone secreted by the corpus luteum after ovulation that prepares the uterine lining to nourish an embryo.

progestin synthetic hormone that has similar action as progesterone.

prolactin pituitary hormone that stimulates breast milk production; excessive amounts can interfere with ovulation.

proliferative phase phase of the menstrual cycle in which, under the influence of estrogen, the endometrium grows thicker in preparation for the implantation of the embryo.

prostate male gland that surrounds the first portion of the urethra near the bladder and secretes a liquid that stimulates sperm movement.

retroflexed uterus anatomic abnormality in which the uterus tilts backward toward the spine and folds inward upon itself.

retrograde ejaculation condition in which semen flows backward into the bladder instead of forward into the urethra.

retroverted uterus (tipped) anatomic abnormality in which the uterus tilts backward toward the spine.

salpingitis inflammation of the Fallopian tubes.

scrotum bag-like structure of skin and muscle that contains the testes.

secondary infertility infertility in a man or a woman who had previously had a biological child.

selective reduction intentional induced termination of one or more gestational sacs, usually in a multiple pregnancy.

semen fluid containing glandular secretions and sperm discharged at ejaculation.

semen analysis microscopic study of fresh ejaculate to determine quantity and quality of sperm.

seminiferous tubules long, tube-like structures in the testicles where sperm are formed.

sexual intercourse sexual union.

sexually transmitted diseases variety of infections, including syphilis, gonorrhea, chlamydia, herpes, and AIDS, contracted through sexual activities.

Sims-Huhner test see postcoital test.

sonogram see ultrasonography.

sperm the male reproductive cell or gamete.

sperm agglutination test microscopic study to determine if sperm clump together, which impedes their ability to swim.

sperm analysis see semen analysis.

spermatogenesis sperm production in the seminiferous tubules.

spermatozoa sperm.

sperm bank places where sperm are cryopreserved and stored for future therapeutic inseminations.

sperm count number of sperm in an ejaculate.

spermicide substance that can kill sperm.

sperm morphology sperm shape.

sperm motility ability of sperm to swim forward.

sperm viscosity thickness of the semen.

sperm washing technique to separate sperm from seminal fluid.

spinnbarkheit stretchability of cervical mucus.

split ejaculate method of semen collection in which the first half of the ejaculate, which usually contains the most sperm, is caught in one container, the second in another.

spontaneous abortion see miscarriage.

Stein-Leventhal Syndrome see polycystic ovarian syndrome.

sterility absolute inability to reproduce.

surrogate third-party reproduction method in which a woman agrees to carry a fetus to term for an infertile couple.

surrogate mother see surrogate.

Tay-Sachs disease deadly hereditary disease affecting young children.

TESE see testicular sperm extraction.

testicles male sex glands, located in the scrotum, which produce testosterone and sperm.

testicular biopsy procedures in which a small amount of testicular tissue is removed and then examined for their ability to produce sperm or for presence of cancerous cells.

testicular sperm extraction (TESE) procedure in which sperm are removed directly from the testicular tissue.

testis male sex organ.

testosterone primary male sex hormone.

test-tube baby popular term to describe babies conceived through assisted reproductive technologies.

TET see tubal embryo transfer.

tuboplasty surgical procedure to repair the Fallopian tubes.

therapeutic insemination donor (TID) third-party reproduction method in which sperm from a donor are placed in a woman's cervix or uterus; artificial insemination.

therapeutic insemination husband (TIH) procedure in which male partner's sperm are placed in the cervix or uterus of the female partner.

tubal embryo transfer (TET) assisted reproductive technology method in which an embryo is placed in the Fallopian tubes.

tubal ligation female sterilization procedure; sometimes called having your "tubes tied."

ultrasonography medical test that uses sound waves to visualize an organ.

undescended testes see cryptorchidism.

unexplained infertility (idiopathic infertility) term to describe no explanation for infertility after a couple has gone through complete testing and evaluation.

urinary luteinizing hormone (LH) test   measures luteinizing hormone in the urine and pin-points more accurately the LH surge that precedes ovulation.

urologist   medical doctor, board-certified in the diagnosis and treatment of disorders of the urinary tract and male sex organs.

uterus   part of the female reproductive system that holds and nourishes a fetus until birth; womb.

vagina   part of the female reproductive system that extends from the vulva to the cervix.

vaginal ultrasound   ultrasound test used to determine follicular development and guide egg retrieval.

varicocele   varicose veins in the testicle.

varicocelectomy   procedure to remove varicoceles.

vas deferens   long, tube-like structure, which rises from the epididymis to the ejaculatory duct and through which sperm travel during ejaculation.

vasectomy   male sterilization procedure.

vasography   X-ray of the vas deferens used to find a blockage or leakage of sperm.

venography   see high-resolution scrotal sonography.

washed sperm cells   sperm cells that have had the seminal plasma removed by centrifugation.

ZIFT   see zygote intrafallopian transfer.

zona pellucida   the hard outer surface of the egg, which allows sperm to penetrate it before fertilization can occur.

zygote   fertilized egg; embryo in the early stages of development.

zygote intrafallopian transfer (ZIFT)   assisted reproduction technology in which a zygote is placed into the Fallopian tubes.

Recommended Reading List

Bradstreet, Karen. *Overcoming Inferitlity Naturally.* Woodland Books, 1995.

Carter, Jean W., and Carter, Michael. *Sweet Grapes: How to Stop Being Infertile and Start Living Again.* Perspectives Press, 1989.

Cooper, Susan Lewis, and Glazer, Ellen Sarasohn. *Choosing Assisted Reproduction: Social, Emotional and Ethical Considerations.* Perspectives Press, 1998.

Cooper, Susan Lewis, and Glazer, Ellen Sarasohn. *Beyond Infertility: A Guide to the New Reproductive Options.* Lexington Books, 1994.

Gilman, Lois. *The Adoption Resource Book.* Third Edition. HarperCollins, 1992.

Glazer, Ellen Sarasohn. *The Long-Awaited Stork: A Guide to Parenting After Infertility.* Lexington Books, 1990.

Goldstein, Marc, Fuerst, Mark, and Berger, Gary S. *The Couples's Guide to Fertility.* Main Street Books, 1995.

Greil, Arthur L. *Not Yet Pregnant: Infertilie Couples in Contemporary America.* Rutgers University Press, 1991.

Jansen, Robert. *Overcoming Infertility: A Compassionate Resource for Getting Pregnant.* W. H. Freeman, *1997.*

Lauersen, Niels. H., and Bouchez, Colette. *Getting Pregnant.* Fawcett Books, 1992.

Liebmann-Smith, Joan. *In Pursuit of Pregnancy.* Newmarket Press, 1989.

Marrs, Richard, Blosch, Lisa Friedman, and Silverman, Kathy Kirtland. *Dr. Marr's Fertility Book.* Dell Publishing, 1998.

Marsh, Margaret, and Wanda Ronner. *The Empty Cradle: Infertility in America from Colonial Times to the Present.* Johns Hopkins University Press. 1996.

May, Elaine Tyler. *Barren In the Promised Land: Childless Americans and the Pursuit of Happiness.* Basic Books, 1995.

Meldrum, David, and Melina, Lois Ruskai. *Making Sense of Adoption.* Harper & Row, 1989.

Menning, Barbara Eck. *Infertility: A Guide for the Childless Couple.* Prentice Hall, 1977.

Noble, Elizabeth. *Having Your Baby by Donor Insemination.* Houghton Mifflin, 1987.

Robin, Peggy. *How to Be a Successful Fertiltiy Patient.* William Morrow and Company, Inc., 1993.

Rosenberg, Helane S. and Epstein, Yakov M. *Getting Pregnant When Your Thought You Couldn't.* Warner Books, 1993.

Sher, Jonathon. *Preventing Miscarriage—The Good News.* Harper Perennial, 1991.

Shulgold, Barbara, and Sipiora, Lynn. *Dear Barbara, Dear Lynne: The True Story of Two Women in Search of Motherhood.* Addison-Wesley, 1992.

Silber, Sherman J. *How to Get Pregnant with the New Technology.* Warner Books, 1998.

Stangel, John J. *The New Fertility and Conception: The Essential Guide for Childless Couples.* 1993.

Vercollone, Carol Frost, Heidi Moss, and Robert Moss. *Helping the Stork: The Choices and Challanges of Donor Insemination,* 1997.

Whitworth, Belinda. *Infertility the Natural Way.* Element Books, 1996.

Zoldbrod, Aline P. *Men Women, and Infertility: Intervention and Treatment Strategies.* Lexington Books, 1993.

Resource Directory

Medical resources

Academy of Assisted Reproductive Technology
    Professionals
611 East Wells
Milwaukee, WI 53202
414-276-4143
Fax: 414-276-3349
E-mail: tvalerine@reproduction.net
Web Site: www.reproduction.net

American Association of Gynecologic
    Laparoscopists
13021 East Florence Avenue
Santa Fe Springs, CA 90670-4505
562-946-8774
800-554-2245 (AAGL)
Fax: 562-946-0073
E-mail: generalmail@aagl.com
Web Site: www.aagl.com

American Association of Tissue Banks (AATB)
1350 Beverly Road
Suite 220A
McLean, VI 22101
703-27-9582
Fax: 703-356-2198
E-mail: aatb@aatb.org

American College of Obstetricians and
    Gynecologists (ACOG)
409 12th Street SW
Washington, DC 20024-2188
202-638-5577

American Society of Andrology (ASA)
74 New Montgomery
Suite 230
San Franciso, CA 94105
415-764-4823
Fax: 415-764-4915
E-mail: asa@hp-assoc.com

American Society for Reproductive Medicine
    (ASRM) (formerly The American Fertility
    Society)
1209 Montgomery Highway
Burmingham, AL 35216-2809
205-978-5000
Web site: www.asrm.org

American Urological Association (AUA)
1120 North Charles Street
Baltimore, MD 21201
301-727-1100

College of American Pathologists (CAP)
325 Waukegan
Northfield, IL 60093
800-323-4000

DES Action, USA (East Coast)
Long Island Jewish Medical Center
New Hyde Park, NY 11040
516-775-3450

DES Action, USA (West Coast)
1615 Broadway
Suite 510
Oakland, CA 94612
510-465-4011

Endocrine Society
4350 East West Highway
Suite 500
Bethseda, MD 20814
301-941-0200
Fax: 301-941-0259
Web Site: www.endo-society.org

Endometriosis Association
8585 North 76th Place
Milwaukee, WI 53223
800-992-3636 (ENDO)

Ferre Institute
258 Genesee St
Suite 302
Utica, NY 13502
315-724-4348
Fax: 315-724-1360
E-mail: FerreInf@aol.com

Infertility Helpline: 800-860-4134

InterNational Council on Infertility Information
    Dissemination (INCIID)
PO Box 6836
Arlington, VA 22206
Phone: 520-544-9548
Fax: 703-379-1593
E-mail: INCIIDinfo@inciid.org
Web site: www.inciid.org

National Society of Genetic Counselors
233 Canterbury Drive
Wallingford, PA 19086
215-872-7608

Organon Inc. (The IVF-Pals Hotline)
West Orange, NJ 07052
800-IVF-PALS

Planned Parenthood Federation of American
810 Seventh Avenue
New York, NY 10019
212-541-7800

Serono Symposia, U.S.A.
100 Longwater Circle
Norwell, MA 02061
800-283-8088
Web site: www.infertilityresource.com

Society for Assisted Reproductive Technology
    (SART)
1209 Montgomery Highway
Birmingham, Al 35216
205-978-5000
E-mail: asrm@asrm.com

Society for Reproductive Surgeons (SRS)
1209 Montgomery Highway
Birmingham, Al 35216
205-978-5000
E-mail: asrm.@asrm.com

Alternative and complementary medicine resources

American Association of Acupuncture and Oriental
  Medicine
4101 Lake Boon Trail
Suite 201
Raleigh, NC 27607-6518

American Association of Oriental Medicine
433 Front St.
Catasauqua PA 18032
610-264-2768
Web site: www.aoom.org

American Association of Naturopathic Physicians
601 Valley Street, #105
Seattle, WA 98109
206-298-0126
Fax: 206-298-0129
E-mail: 74602.3715@compuserve.com
Web site: www.naturopathic.org

American Botanical Council
PO Box 201660
Austin, TX 78720-1660
Web site: www.herbalgram.org

National Acupuncture and Oriental Medicine
Alliance
14637 Starr Road SE
Olalla, WA 98359
253-851-6896
Web site: www.acuall.org

National Center for Homeopathy
801 N. Fairfax Street
Suite 306
Alexandria, VA 22314
Web site: www.healthy.net

National Commission for the Certification of
    Acupuncturists
1424 16th St NW
Suite 501
Washington, DC 20036
202-232-1404

Office of Alternative Medicine Clearinghouse
PO Box 8218
Silver Spring, MD 20907-8218
888-644-6226
Fax: 301-495-4957
Web site: almed.od.nih.gov

Consumer information organizations
RESOLVE
1310 Broadway
Somerville, MA 02144-1731
Helpline: 617-623-0744
Business line: 617-623-1156
Web site: www.resolve.org

Adoption
Adoptees Liberty Movement Association
PO Box 154
Washington Bridge Station
New York, New York 10033
212-581-1568

Adoptive Families of America (formally OURS, Inc.)
3333 Highway 100 North
Minneapolis, MN 55422
612-535-4829
612-434-4930

American Adoption Congress
1000 Connecticut Avenue NW
Washington, DC 20036
800-274-6736

Child Welfare League of America
440 First Street NW
Washington, DC 20001
202-628-2952

Committee for Single Adoptive Parents
PO Box 15084
Chevy Chase, MD 20815

International Alliance for Children, Inc.
2 Ledge Lane
New Milford, CT
203-354-354-3417

Latin American Parents Association (LAPA)
PO Box 72
Seaford, NY 11783
516-783-6942

National Adoption Center
1218 Chestnut Street
Philadelphia, PA 19107
215-925-0200

National Adoption Information Clearinghouse
11426 Rockville Pike
Rockville, MD 20852
301-231-6512

National Council for Adoption
1930 17th Street NW
Washington, DC
202-328-1200

National Resource Center for Special Needs
    Adoption
16250 Northland Drive
Suite 120
Southfield, MI 48075
313-433-7080

North American Council on Adoptable Children
    (NACAC)
970 Raymond Street, Suite 106
St. Paul, MN 55114-1149
612-644-3036
Fax: 612-644-9848

Single Mothers by Choice
Box 7788
FDR Station
New York, NY 10150

Miscarriages

Compassionate Friends
PO Box 3696
Oakbrook, IL 60522-3696
708-990-0020

Miscellaneous

Lact-Aid International, Inc.
PO Box 10066
Athen, TN 37303
615-744-9090

La Leche League International
PO Box 1209
Franklin Park, IL 60131-8209

Center for Reproductive Alternatives
3333 Vincent Road
Suite 222
Pleasant Hill, CA 94523
415-930-6220

Third-party reproduction

American Surrogacy Center
638 Church Street NE
Marietta, GA 30063
770-426-1107
E-mail: TASC@surrogacy.com
Web site: www.surrogacy.com

Biogenics Corporation
1130 Rt. 22 West
PO Box 1290
Mountside, NJ 07092
908-654-8836
Fax: 908-232-2114

California Cryobank, Inc.
1019 Gayley Avenue
Los Angeles, CA 90024
800-231-3373
Fax: 310-208-8477
Web site: www.cryobank.com

Center for Surrogate Parenting & Egg Donation,
    Inc.
8383 Wilshire Blvd
Suite 750
Beverly Hill, CA 90211
213-655-1974
Fax: 213-852-1310
E-mail: Centersp@aol.com
Web sites: www.centersp@aol.com;
    www.eggdonor.com

Cryogenic Laboratories, Inc.
1944 Lexington Avenue North
Roseville, Minnesota 55113
612-489-8000
Fax: 612-489-8989
E-mail: cryolabinc@aol.com

Fairfax Cryobank, A Division of The Genetics & IVF
    Institutes
3015 Williams Drive
Suite 110
Fairfax, VA 22031
703-698-3976
Fax: 703-698-3933

IDANT Laboratories
350 Fifth Avenue
Suite 7120
New York, NY 10118
212-244-0555
Fax: 212-244-0806
E-mail: info@daxor-idant.com
Web site: www.daxor-idant.com

Organization of Parents Through Surrogacy
    (OPTS)
PO Box 213
Wheeling, IL 60090

Park Avenue Fertility Group
1080 Park Avenue
New York, NY 10128
212-289-5866
Fax: 212-289-2005

Surrogate Mother Program, Inc.
220 West 93rd Street
New York, NY 10025
212-496-1070

Surrogate Parent Program
11110 Ohio Avenue
Suite 202
Los Angeles, CA 90025
310-473-8961

Woman To Woman Fertility Center, Inc.
3201 Danville Blvd.
Suite 160
Danville, CA 94507
925-820-9495
Fax: 925-820-3885
E-mail: wwfc@compuserve.com

Xytex Corporation
1110 Emmett St
Augusta, GA 30904
800-277-3210
Fax: 706-736-9720
E-mail: xytex@xytex.com

Child-free living

Childless by Choice
PO Box 695
Leavenworth, WA 98826
509-763-2112
Website: www.now2000.com/cbc

National Organization for Nonparents
806 Reistertown Road
Baltimore, MD 21208

Other useful web sites

Centers for Disease Control and Prevention:
Web site: www.cdc.gov

Child of My Dreams Resource Center: www.
child-dream.com

Fertilitext: www.fertilitext.ogan

Fertilethoughts: www.fertilethoughts.net/
infertility/index.html

National Institutes of Health: www.nih.gov

Medline: www.medline.web.aol.com

TASC: The American Surrogacy Center, Inc.:
www.surrogacy.com

U.S. Food and Drug Administration: www.fda.gov

Mail order pharmacies

Eveready Drugs, Ltd.
1229 Third Avenue
New York, NY 10021
800-424-3378
Fax: 516-242-4113
Web site: www.evereadydrugs.com

IVP Phamaeutical Care, Inc.
2833 Trinity Square Drive
Suite 105
Carrollton, TX 75006
800-424-9002
Fax: 800-874-9179
E-mail: sales@ivpcare.com
Web site: www.ivpcare.com

MDRx Encino Pharmacy
16500 Ventura Blvd
Encino, CA 91436
818-788-3784 (DRUG)
Fax: 818-788-0607

MDRx Pharmaceutical Care
16500 Ventura Blvd.
Encino, CA 91436
800-515-3784 (DRUG)
Fax: 818-788-0607
E-mail: info@mdrusa.com
Web site: www.mdrusa.com

MDRx Westwood Center Pharmacy
10921 Whilshire Blvd
Los Angeles, CA 90024
310-208-6666
Fax: 310-824-0056

Park Avenue Chemist, Ldt.
1080 Park Avenue
New York, NY 10128
212-289-5866
Fax: 212-289-2005

Schraft's Pharmacy
1114 Springfield Avenue
Irvington, NJ 07111
973-373-1651
Fax: 973-373-2664

Stadtlanders Pharmacy
600 Penn Center Boulevard
Pittsburgh, PA 15235-5810
800-238-7828
Web site: stadlander.com

Publications and publishers

Fertility and Sterility
American Society for Reproductive Medicine
1209 Montgomery Highway
Birmingham, Al 35216
205-978-5000
Fax: 205-978-5005
E-mail: asrm@asrm.com
Web site: www.asrm.com/profession/fertility/
fspage.html

Fertility Weekly
1087 Crooked Creek Road SE
Eatonton, GA 31024
800-705-7185
Fax: 706-484-1813
E-mail: kkey@hendersonnet.atl.ga.us
Web site: www.holonet.not/homepage/fwabut.htm

INCIID Insights
International Council on Infertility Information
Dissemination
PO Box 91363
Tuscon, AZ 85752-1363
520-544-9548
Fax 520-509-5251
E-mail: INCIIDinfo@aol.com
Web site: tieswww.inciid.org

Newsletter of RESOLVE
1310 Broadway
Somerville, MA 02114
617-623-0744
Fax: 617-623-0252
E-mail: resolveinc@aol.com
Web site: www.resolve.org

Perspectives Press
PO Box 90318
Indianapolis, IN 46290-0318
317-872-3055
E-mail: ppress@iquest.net
Web site: www.perspectivespress.com

Important Documents

Flow sheet of infertility investigation

Name:_____
Chart # _____

Duration of Infertility:

    Primary or Secondary

Past History (Pertinent Facts)

    Obstet: _____

    Surgical: _____

    Childhood illnesses
    (allergies): _____

    Nutrition: _____

Menstrual History: _____

    Interval: _____

    Amenorrhea: _____

Sexual History: Frequency of Intercourse_____

General Physical Exam

Height_____   Weight_____

    Abnormalities:_____

Pelvic Exam:_____

    Abnormalities:_____

Basal Temperature:_____

    Monophasic: _____

    Biphasic:_____

Equivocal: _____

Ovarian Function: _____

   Endometrial Biopsy: _____

   Serum progesterone:_____

   Laparoscopic observation: _____

Tubal Patency: _____

   Rubins Test: _____

   Hysterosalpingogram: _____

   Laparoscopy: _____

Uterus: _____

   Hysterogram: _____

   Hysteroscopy: _____

   Abnormalities at laparoscopy: _____

Cervix: _____

   Mucus: _____

Normal _____   Abnormal _____

   Post Coital Test:_____ No sperm/hpf: _____

   "Shaking" sperm: _____

   Progressive Sperm: _____

   Immunologic (If Indicated): _____

Sample Donor Profile

XYZ LABORATORIES DONOR PROFILE

Donor Code _____

Date of Birth _____

PHYSICAL CHARACTERISTICS

Eye Color _____	Hair Color _____	Hair Type _____
Height _____	Weight _____	Body Type _____
Complexion _____	Racial Group _____	Blood Group
Ethnic Origin _____	Religion _____	and RH _____

PERSONAL AND EDUCATIONAL BACKGROUND

Marital Status _____

Children _____

Proven Fertility _____

Educational Status and Field of Study _____

Occupation _____

Interests/Hobbies _____

Special Skills/Talents _____

DONOR/FAMILY MEDICAL HISTORY

For each item below, there is no known history of the condition unless otherwise noted.

__Hay Fever	__Drug/Alcohol Abuse	__Early Death (before 50)
__Asthma	__Blood Disease	__Mature Onset Diabetes
__Allergies	__Thyroid Disease	__Congenital Hip
__Cancer	__Cardiac Disease	Problems

__Gout	__Schizophrenia	__Congenital Heart Disease
__Epilepsy	__Mental Disorders	__Arthritis (before 50)
__Hepatitis	__Kidney Disease	__Premature Senility
__Blindness	__Eye Disorders	__Cataracts (before 40)
__Infertility	__Cystic Fibrosis	__Deafness (before 50)
__Club Feet	__Down's Syndrome	__Miscarriages or Stillbirths
__Thalassemia	__Tay Sachs Disease	
__Herpes	__Venereal Disease	__Serious Birth Defects
__A.I.D.S.	__Chemical Exposure	__Sickle Cell Trait
__Radiation Exposure	__Cleft Lip/Palate	

Key to Codes:

D: Donor   **M:** Mother   **F:** Father   **B:** Brother   **S:** Sister

A: Aunt   **U:** Uncle   **C:** Cousin

MGM/F: Maternal Grandmother/Grandfather

PGM/F: Paternal Grandmother/Grandfather

Semen Analysis Report

SEMEN ANALYSIS REPORT: BASIC ANALYSIS

Physician _____

Office_____

Specimen No. _____

Patient Name _____

Spouse's Name _____

Patient SSN _____

Spouse's SSN _____

Andrology Service(s)

Requested _____

Specimen

Date Collected_____   Time Collected_____

Time arrived in lab _____

Complete _____

Incomplete _____

If incomplete, portion lost_____

Location of

collection _____

Date of last

emission _____

Gross Examination	**Reference Values**
Volume_____	2.0-5.0 mL
pH_____	Alkaline
Color_____	Gray-white
Liquefaction _____	Complete by 20 min.
Viscosity_____	Completely liquid

Microscopic Examination

Particulate Debris _____	Not excessive
Agglutinated Clumps _____	Not excessive
Mucus_____	Not excessive
Sperm motility (time:_____)	Over 50% progressive

Total Progressive _____%

Quick Progressive _____%

Sluggish Progressive _____%

Non Progressive_____%

Sperm viability _____% dead   Less than 35%
                                     dead

Sperm concentration   20-200 million/mL

   1._____dilution: _____million/mL

   2._____dilution: _____million/mL

Total progressive   Sperm per ejaculate

_____million   >50 million

Sperm morphology

   Normal Oval _____%

   Abnormal _____%

   Small Oval Heads _____%

   Large Oval Heads _____%

   Amorphous Heads _   _____%

   Neck Defects: _____%

   Round Heads _____%

   Tapered Heads _____%

   Cytoplasmic Droplets: _____%

   Double Heads or Tails: _____%

   Coiled Tails: _____%

   Other Abnormal Forms: _____%

   Round Cells: _____%

   WBCs: _____%

   Immature Germ Cells: _____%

Comments:

_____

_____

_____

_____

_____

_____

A

The *Unofficial Guide*™ Reader Questionnaire

If you would like to express your opinion about infertility or this guide, please complete this questionnaire and mail it to:

The *Unofficial Guide*™ Reader Questionnaire
Macmillan Lifestyle Group
1633 Broadway, floor 7
New York, NY 10019-6785

Gender: ___ M ___ F

Age: ___ Under 30 ___ 31–40 ___ 41–50
___ Over 50

Education: ___ High school ___ College
___ Graduate/Professional

What is your occupation?

_____

How did you hear about this guide?
___ Friend or relative
___ Newspaper, magazine, or Internet
___ Radio or TV
___ Recommended at bookstore
___ Recommended by librarian
___ Picked it up on my own
___ Familiar with the *Unofficial Guide*™ travel series

Did you go to the bookstore specifically for a book on infertility? Yes ___ No ___

Have you used any other *Unofficial Guides*™?
Yes ___ No ___

If Yes, which ones?

_____
_____
_____

What other book(s) on infertility have you purchased?

_____
_____
_____

Was this book:
___ more helpful than other(s)
___ less helpful than other(s)

Do you think this book was worth its price?
Yes ___ No ___

Did this book cover all topics related to infertility adequately? Yes ___ No ___

Please explain your answer:

_____
_____
_____

Were there any specific sections in this book that were of particular help to you? Yes ___ No ___

Please explain your answer:

_____
_____
_____

On a scale of 1 to 10, with 10 being the best rating, how would you rate this guide? ___

What other titles would you like to see published in the _Unofficial Guide_™ series?

_____
_____

Are _Unofficial Guides_™ readily available in your area? Yes ___ No ___

Other comments:

_____
_____
_____
_____

Get the inside scoop...with the Unofficial Guides™!

The Unofficial Guide to Alternative Medicine
ISBN: 0-02-862526-9 Price: $15.95

The Unofficial Guide to Buying a Home
ISBN: 0-02-862461-0 Price: $15.95

The Unofficial Guide to Childcare
ISBN: 0-02-862457-2 Price: $15.95

The Unofficial Guide to Conquering Impotence
ISBN: 0-02-862870-5 Price: $15.95

The Unofficial Guide to Coping with Menopause
ISBN: 0-02-862694-X Price: $15.95

The Unofficial Guide to Cosmetic Surgery
ISBN: 0-02-862522-6 Price: $15.95

The Unofficial Guide to Dating Again
ISBN: 0-02-862454-8 Price: $15.95

The Unofficial Guide to Dieting Safely
ISBN: 0-02-862521-8 Price: $15.95

The Unofficial Guide to Divorce
ISBN: 0-02-862455-6 Price: $15.95

The Unofficial Guide to Having a Baby
ISBN: 0-02-862695-8 Price: $15.95

The Unofficial Guide to Investing
ISBN: 0-02-862458-0 Price: $15.95

The Unofficial Guide to Investing in Mutual Funds
ISBN: 0-02-862920-5 Price: $15.95

The Unofficial Guide to Planning Your Wedding
ISBN: 0-02-862459-9 Price: $15.95

All books in the *Unofficial Guide*™ series are available at your local bookseller, or by calling 1-800-428-5331.

About the Authors

Joan Liebmann-Smith, Ph.D. is a medical sociologist and an award-winning medical writer. Her articles have appeared in such publications as *American Health, Longevity, Ms., Redbook, Self* and *Vogue*, and she is the author of another book on infertility, *In Pursuit of Pregnancy* (Newmarket, 1987, 1989).

Dr. Liebmann-Smith is a past co-president of RESOLVE, NYC and a past board member of RESOLVE, INC. She is on the board of the National Council on Women's Health and is a research scientist at the American Health Foundation.

Jacqueline Nardi Egan is a medical journalist. She specializes in writing educational programs for physicians, allied health professionals, patients, and consumers. She has been the editor of several specialty medical publications and a medical editor of *Family Health* magazine.

John S. Stangel, MD, Clinical Director of Reproductive Medicine, Department of Obstetrics & Gynecology and Women's Health, Montefiore Medical Center, The University Hospital for the Albert Einstein College of Medicine, is board certified in Reproductive Endocrinology and Infertility. He has been the Medical Director of IVF America Program–Westchester in a Clinical Associate Professor in the Department of Obstetrics and Gynecology at New York Medical College at Metropolitan Hospital, and at the Westchester County Medical.

Dr. Stangel is a charter member of both the Society of Reproductive Endocrinologists and the Society of Reproductive Surgeons.

Dr. Stangel is the editor and contributing author of the textbook, *Infertility Surgery.* He also authored *The New Fertility and Conception.*